Respiratory Function of the Lung and Its Control

MODERN CONCEPTS IN MEDICAL PHYSIOLOGY

A MACMILLAN SERIES

Lysle H. Peterson, M.D., Consulting Editor

Fred S. Grodins, M.D., Ph.D.

PROFESSOR AND CHAIRMAN, DEPARTMENT OF BIOMEDICAL ENGINEERING,
AND PROFESSOR OF PHYSIOLOGY,
UNIVERSITY OF SOUTHERN CALIFORNIA

Stanley M. Yamashiro, Ph.D.

ASSOCIATE PROFESSOR OF BIOMEDICAL ENGINEERING,
UNIVERSITY OF SOUTHERN CALIFORNIA

Respiratory Function of the Lung and Its Control

Macmillan Publishing Co., Inc.
New York

Collier Macmillan Canada, Ltd.
Toronto

Baillière Tindall
London

Copyright © 1978, Fred S. Grodins

Printed in the United States of America

All rights reserved. No part of this book may be reproduced or transmitted in any form or by any means, electronic or mechanical, including photocopying, recording, or any information storage and retrieval system, without permission in writing from the Publisher.

Macmillan Publishing Co., Inc.
866 Third Avenue, New York, New York 10022

Collier Macmillan Canada, Ltd.

Baillière Tindall · London

Library of Congress Cataloging in Publication Data

Grodins, Fred S
  Respiratory function of the lung and its control.

  (Modern concepts in medical physiology)
  Bibliography: p.
  Includes index.
  1. Respiration—Regulation. 2. Lungs. I. Yamashiro, Stanley M., (date) joint author. II. Title. [DNLM: 1. Lung—Physiology. 2. Respiratory function tests. WF102 G873r]
QP123.G76   612'.2   77-18280
ISBN 0-02-348190-0
ISBN 0-02-348120-X pbk.

Baillière Tindall SBN   07020-07072

Printing: 1 2 3 4 5 6 7 8   Year: 8 9 0 1 2 3 4

Preface

THIS BOOK HAS EVOLVED from hand-out lecture notes used for many years in teaching respiratory physiology to medical students and to graduate and senior undergraduate students in physiology, biology, and biomedical engineering. It should also be of interest to specialists in anesthesiology, pulmonary medicine, and respiratory therapy. The text is organized to stress the analysis-synthesis dual approach essential in modern systems physiology. An introductory survey describes the components of the system and their organization into a metabolic servomechanism that meets metabolic demands for oxygen and CO_2 transport while regulating against hypoxia and disturbances in acid-base balance. After a brief review of the gas laws and their applications in respiration (Chapter 2), the next four chapters analyze the components in detail: "The Ventilatory Apparatus" (Chapter 3), "The Pulmonary Gas Exchanger" (Chapter 4), "Tissue Gas Exchange" (Chapter 5), and "Blood Buffers and Acid-Base Balance" (Chapter 6). Chapter 7 ("Control of Pulmonary Ventilation") is a synthesis, using the theme of control and communication (homeostasis, cybernetics) to emphasize the interactions between the several components as they respond to physiologic and pathologic demands in health and disease.

Many sources, both written and unwritten, have contributed to this effort over some 30 years. It is impossible to acknowledge all of them, but one whose influence is clearly evident throughout is John S. Gray, the former teacher and colleague of one of us (FSG) at Northwestern University Medical School from 1947–1967. We dedicate this book to him.

Fred S. Grodins
Stanley M. Yamashiro

Contents

1	Introductory Survey of the Respiratory System	1
2	Gas Laws and Applications	8
3	The Ventilatory Apparatus	17
4	The Pulmonary Gas Exchanger	46
5	Tissue Gas Exchange	86
6	Blood Buffers and Acid-Base Balance	95
7	Control of Pulmonary Ventilation	108
	Index	143

Respiratory Function of the Lung and Its Control

CHAPTER 1

Introductory Survey of the Respiratory System

THE OVERALL BEHAVIOR of the respiratory system in man is an expression of the integrated interaction of many different unit processes. To understand this behavior, we must examine both the unit processes and their interactions. That the latter are at least as important as the former is clear from the fact that a single set of unit processes may be "programmed" to perform a great variety of overall tasks (e.g., in the analog or digital computer). An approach that emphasizes an understanding of the overall behavior of complex systems in terms of interacting unit processes has been formally recognized in recent years under the name *Systems Analysis*. In a sense, this is a misnomer, for the really new feature is the emphasis on synthesis. Analysis, after all, has been with us since the dawn of science. An important type of interaction that occurs frequently in biologic systems is negative feedback, and it is rewarding to examine such systems in the framework of control theory. This is the approach we shall adopt in our study of respiration.

How small should our unit processes be? There is no unique answer to this question except to say that they should be small enough to contribute to useful understanding but not so small as to introduce unnecessary complication and confusion at the overall level of primary interest. This may not seem to be a very satisfactory answer, but fortunately we are reasonably successful at making proper intuitive choices in practice. Thus none of us would try to understand the overall behavior of an automobile in terms of the elementary nuclear particles of which it is composed, even though we acknowledge their ultimate relevance. To the busy clinician pressed for time and committed to prompt action, explicit analysis of disease in terms of any unit process smaller than the "whole man" may seem an unnecessary luxury. Nevertheless, we are certain that he does make such an analysis implicitly and that it contributes significantly to sound clinical judgment.

What are the overall functions of the respiratory system? The most obvious one is oxygen procurement and carbon dioxide elimination at rates required by tissue metabolism. Since no significant oxygen stores exist in the body, a continuous external supply is essential for survival. Thus man can live weeks without food, days without water, but only a few minutes without oxygen. In exercise, tissue oxygen requirements may increase tenfold, and this demand must be promptly met. To do so requires a cooperative effort by the respiratory (external procurement) and cardiovascular (internal transport and distribution) systems, which are inseparably coupled in this task of metabolic gas transport and exchange. Not only must gross oxygen exchange rate be adequate but efficient tissue utilization requires that it be accomplished at sufficiently high levels of internal oxygen concentration. The nervous system is particularly sensitive to low oxygen concentration, and, in most common types of hypoxia, it is the internal concentration rather than the gross exchange rate that is low. Considerations of this sort lead us to look at the O_2 procurement and CO_2 elimination functions of respiration from another point of view, one that lies at the heart of physiology, i.e., homeostasis, or regulation.

Thus, instead of saying that the function of respiration is to procure O_2 and eliminate CO_2 at rates required by tissue metabolism, we can say that its function is to regulate arterial blood concentrations of O_2, CO_2, and H^+ within prescribed limits. This view is a much more powerful and general one and implies the existence of active control processes that would not otherwise be necessary. For example, a single cell in direct contact with its external environment through a passive membrane could procure O_2 and eliminate CO_2 by simple diffusion at rates required by its metabolism, provided its internal O_2 concentration were allowed to fall and its internal CO_2 concentration to rise sufficiently to establish the necessary concentration gradients. But this is a very restricted process, for internal P_{O_2} obviously cannot fall below zero and internal P_{CO_2} cannot rise too high without producing fatal increases in acidity. If, on the other hand, we had an active membrane that could "pump" O_2 into and CO_2 out of the cell, and if its pumping rates depended in appropriate ways upon internal O_2 and CO_2 concentrations, we could "automatically" match exchange rates to metabolism over a much wider range with minimal changes in internal concentrations. Not only could we do that, but we could also automatically guard against other kinds of disturbances that might threaten internal concentrations, e.g., increased CO_2 in the external environment, or increased production of "fixed acids" by a faulty metabolic machinery.

It turns out that we can bring these two views together in the context of control and servomechanism theory. Thus we can say that what we have here is a metabolic servomechanism designed to match pulmonary and metabolic gas exchange rates without alteration of internal chemical concentrations by active manipulation of pulmonary ventilation, and whose error-correcting feedback signals are provided by the concentrations of O_2, CO_2, and H^+ in arterial blood. As we shall see in later chapters, it is much easier to identify the error-correcting chemical feedback signals than it is to find the "metabolic command signal" that should provide the servosystem's primary input.

What basic structures and unit processes do we encounter in exploring the details of our respiratory metabolic servomechanism? It is not difficult to list them proceeding from the "outside in":

1. There is a mechanism for the bulk transfer of gas between the external atmosphere and the internal gas phase in the lung alveoli. This utilizes a "bellows" technique, i.e., the alternate expansion and compression of a hollow chamber in communication with the atmosphere. The energy to operate the bellows comes from the respiratory muscles. We shall collectively call all of the structures concerned the *ventilatory apparatus* and the unit process *pulmonary ventilation*.

2. There is a mechanism for the transfer of gases between the internal gas phase and the blood in the pulmonary capillaries. The mechanism is one of passive diffusion which follows well-known physicochemical laws. We shall call the structures concerned the *pulmonary diffusion apparatus* and the unit process *pulmonary diffusion*.

3. There is an internal transport medium (the blood) so structured that it can carry sufficient O_2 and CO_2 to meet tissue needs within existing constraints imposed by ambient P_{O_2}, pulmonary ventilation rates, blood flow rates, and permissible internal concentrations of H^+. We shall call this medium the *blood chemical apparatus* and the unit process *blood chemical processing*.

4. There is an internal pumping and distribution system to move blood from lungs to tissues and back again. We shall call this structural component the *cardiovascular system* and the unit process *circulation*.

5. There is a mechanism for transferring O_2 and CO_2 between blood in the systemic capillaries and the tissues. Again, it is accomplished by passive diffusion. We call this the *tissue diffusion apparatus* and the unit process *tissue diffusion*.

6. Finally, we have the metabolizing tissues themselves which consume oxygen at a rate, $\dot{V}_{O_2}$ L/min, and produce CO_2 at a rate, $\dot{V}_{CO_2}$ L/min. The ratio of these two tissue rates, $\dot{V}_{CO_2}/\dot{V}_{O_2}$, is called the "respiratory quotient," RQ. We shall call this component the *metabolic system* and the unit process *tissue metabolism*.

We can summarize the system so far described by tracing the flow of O_2 and CO_2 through the "hardware diagram" in Figure 1-1. Numerical values for important respiratory quantities are given in the diagram for a resting man breathing atmospheric air at sea level. The ventilatory apparatus on the left is connected to the metabolizing tissues on the right by the cardiovascular system that lies between.

Atmospheric air with an oxygen partial pressure ($P_{I_{O_2}}$) of 160 mm Hg and a CO_2 partial pressure ($P_{I_{CO_2}}$) of essentially zero enters the lung alveoli during inspiration. Here it is exposed to mixed venous blood entering the pulmonary capillaries with a $P_{V_{O_2}}$ of 43 mm Hg and a $P_{V_{CO_2}}$ of 47 mm Hg. Passive diffusion of O_2 from air to blood and of CO_2 from blood to air thus takes place across the alveolocapillary membrane until equilibrium is reached at a P_{O_2} of 103 mm Hg and a P_{CO_2} of 40 mm Hg. The equilibrated air, which now contains less O_2 and more CO_2 than inspired air, is called "alveolar air" ($P_{A_{O_2}} = 103$; $P_{A_{CO_2}} = 40$), and the equilibrated blood, which now contains more O_2 and less CO_2 than mixed venous blood, is called "end capillary blood" ($P_{ec_{O_2}} = 103$; $P_{ec_{CO_2}} = 40$). The alveolar air now leaves the lung during expiration, mixes with air of inspired composition that remained in the "dead space" (i.e., the conducting, nonexchanging airways) at the end of the previous inspiration, and becomes expired air with a composition intermediate between that of inspired and alveolar air ($P_{E_{O_2}} = 115$; $P_{E_{CO_2}} = 29.5$). End capillary blood leaving the lung normally mixes with a small amount of blood of venous composition that bypasses the lungs through anatomical shunt pathways (chiefly the bronchial circulation), and the mixture is called arterial blood. The properties of the blood chemical processor are such that this small "venous admixture" produces no detectable change in $P_{ec_{CO_2}}$, so that $P_{a_{CO_2}} = P_{ec_{CO_2}} = P_{A_{CO_2}}$; however, it does produce an appreciable drop (8 mm Hg) in $P_{ec_{O_2}}$, so that $P_{a_{O_2}} < P_{ec_{O_2}} = P_{A_{O_2}}$. The left heart pumps the arterial blood to the tissues, which actively consume oxygen ($\dot{V}_{O_2} = 0.275$ L/min) and produce CO_2 ($\dot{V}_{CO_2} = 0.234$ L/min) and in so doing set up diffusion gradients across the tissue-capillary gas exchanger. Passive diffusion of O_2 from blood to tissue and of CO_2 from tissue to blood therefore occurs across the capillary membrane, and the blood leaves the tissue exchanger as mixed venous blood with $P_{V_{O_2}} = 43$ and $P_{V_{CO_2}} = 47$. This blood is pumped back to the pulmonary exchanger and the exchange cycle begins again. In the steady state, the gas exchange rates across the lung, $\dot{V}_{O_2}$, $\dot{V}_{CO_2}$, and their ratio, R (the

INTRODUCTORY SURVEY OF THE RESPIRATORY SYSTEM 5

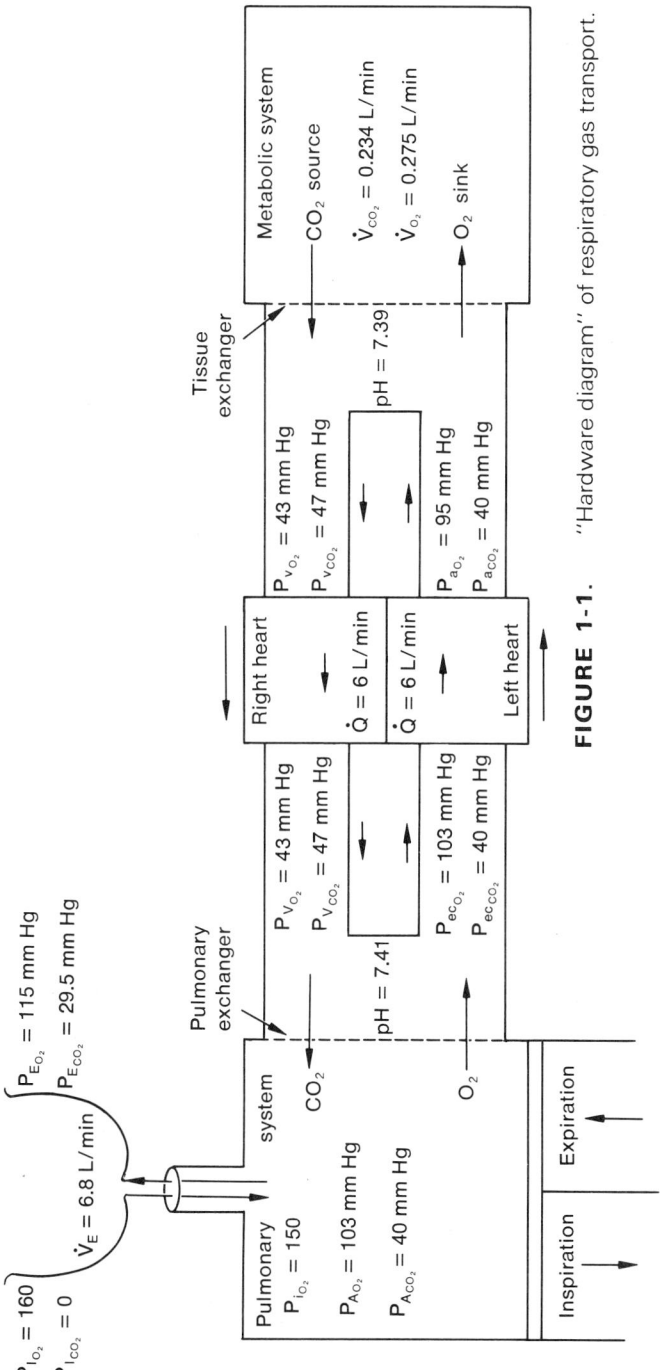

FIGURE 1-1. "Hardware diagram" of respiratory gas transport.

"respiratory exchange ratio"), measured by analysis of inspired and expired air, are equal to the corresponding tissue metabolic rates of O_2 consumption and CO_2 production and their ratio, RQ (the respiratory quotient), in the metabolic system. However, since there is a large storage capacity for CO_2 in the body, transient states may occur during which $\dot{V}_{CO_2}$, and thus R, measured across the lung, are not equal to the metabolic CO_2 production rate and RQ. The value of the metabolic respiratory quotient, RQ, depends only upon the food material being oxidized, ranging from 0.7 for a pure fat substrate to 1.0 for pure carbohydrate, and averaging about 0.85 on a normal mixed diet. However, the expired respiratory exchange ratio, R, will fall below RQ if body CO_2 stores are increasing or rise above it if these stores are decreasing during transient states.

Although both air pumping by the ventilatory apparatus and blood pumping by the heart are cyclic rather than continuous processes, it is customary to average the volumes pumped over a 1-min period and to call this average *pulmonary ventilation* for the lung pump ($\dot{V}_E$ = 6.8 L/min) and "cardiac output" for the heart pump ($\dot{Q}$ = 6.0 L/min). In severe exercise when $\dot{V}_{O_2}$ may rise over tenfold to 3.5 L/min, $\dot{V}_E$ increases to 120 L/min, and $\dot{Q}$ to 35 L/min.

Figure 1-1 is a material flow diagram in which we can conveniently trace the flow of O_2 and CO_2 through the lung-blood-tissue respiratory complex. However, it has nothing to say about the operation of our metabolic servosystem. To examine this, we need a different sort of block diagram and this appears in Figure 1-2.

This diagram conforms in pattern and purpose to a feedback control system. In constructing it, we have assumed that the respira-

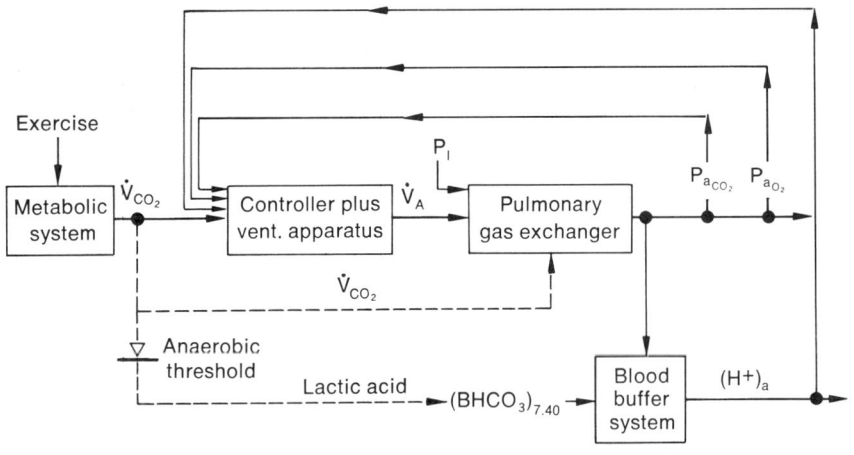

FIGURE 1-2. Diagram of the "Metabolic Servomechanism."

tory system comprises a metabolic servomechanism designed to match pulmonary and metabolic gas exchange rates over a wide range with no change in arterial composition. We have further assumed that it does this by providing the "controller" block with a "command signal" telling it to vary $\dot{V}_E$ in direct proportion to $\dot{V}_{CO_2}$. If the controller does this, then the outputs of the "process," $P_{a_{CO_2}}$, $P_{a_{O_2}}$, and $(H^+)_a$, will remain constant. If it does not, then these outputs will change. Hence, if their values are sensed and "fed back" to the controller, the latter will be informed of its degree of success in matching external gas exchange to metabolic needs and can correct any "error." Because of the nature of its feedback, this system will also act as a regulator to partially correct any deviations in $P_{a_{CO_2}}$, $P_{a_{O_2}}$, and $(H^+)_a$ brought about by such disturbances as CO_2 inhalation, altitude hypoxia, and metabolic acidosis.

In the chapters to follow, we shall seek to understand the operation of this metabolic servosystem through the complementary processes of analysis and synthesis. We shall begin with a brief review of the gas laws, which are essential tools in the study of respiratory physiology.

References

1. Gray, J. S. The multiple factor theory of the control of respiratory ventilation. *Science* **103:** 739–744, 1946.
2. Grodins, F. S. *Control Theory and Biological Systems.* New York: Columbia University Press, 1963.
3. Grodins, F. S. Regulation of pulmonary ventilation. *Physiologist* **7:** 319–333, 1964.
4. Grodins, F. S., and S. M. Yamashiro. Control of ventilation. In: *Lung Biology in Health and Disease* (Executive Editor, Claude Lenfant). Vol. 3: *Bioengineering Aspects of the Lung.* Edited by J. B. West. New York: Marcel Dekker, Inc., 1977, p. 515.
5. Hornbein, T. F., and S. C. Sørensen. The chemical regulation of ventilation. In: *Physiology and Biophysics,* 20th ed., Vol. 2. Edited by T. C. Ruch and H. D. Patton. Philadelphia: W. B. Saunders Company, 1974.
6. Kellog, R. H. Central chemical regulation of respiration. In: *Handbook of Physiology,* Section 3, *Respiration,* Vol. 1. Edited by W. O. Fenn and H. Rahn. Washington, D.C.: American Physiological Society, 1964, p. 507.
7. Lambertsen, C. J. Respiration. In: *Medical Physiology,* 13th ed. Edited by V. B. Mountcastle. St. Louis, Mo.: The C. V. Mosby Company, 1974, p. 58.

CHAPTER 2

Gas Laws and Applications

Ideal Gas

EXPERIMENTALLY, IT HAS BEEN FOUND that all gases behave essentially in the same way provided temperatures are not too low and pressures are not too high. Thus the volume, V, occupied by a mass, m, of any kind of gas depends on the pressure, P, to which the gas is subjected, and on its temperature, T. This interrelationship is neatly summarized by the empirical equation of state of an ideal gas:

$$PV = nRT \tag{1}$$

The quantity, n, refers to the mass in terms of the number of moles (n = m/M, M = molecular weight) and R is the universal gas constant. In physiology, volumes are commonly expressed in liters, pressures in millimeters of mercury or centimeters of water, and temperatures in degrees centigrade (or degrees Kelvin). In this system of units,

$$R = 62.37 \frac{\text{liter} \cdot \text{mm Hg}}{\text{mole} \cdot {}^\circ K}$$

if pressure is measured in millimeters of mercury.

All real gases deviate from ideal gas behavior, especially at high pressures. However, over the physiologic range of pressures, most gases can be adequately described by equation (1). For a fixed mass (or fixed number of moles) and a constant temperature, equation (1) becomes

$$PV = \text{const} \qquad (2)$$

The observation that the product of pressure and volume of a fixed mass of gas at constant temperature is constant was first made by Robert Boyle in 1660. As we shall see later, this equation has many applications in respiratory mechanics.

Dalton's Law

In a mixture of gases, such as occurs in the atmosphere or the lung, the total pressure is equal to the sum of the pressures exerted by its component gases. These separate pressures are called the partial pressures of the components. The partial pressure of each gas in the mixture is the same pressure that would be present if the gas occupied the entire mixture volume alone. Thus each gas in a mixture behaves independently of the others. This fact is known as Dalton's law. The partial pressure, P_g, of a gas is often described as

$$P_g = F_g B \qquad (3)$$

where F_g is the volumetric fraction of the gas and B is the total pressure of the mixture.

Water Vapor

One gas that requires special treatment is water vapor. Unlike the other respiratory gases, water is a liquid at ordinary temperatures. The maximum partial pressure of water in a wet gas at a given temperature is equal to the vapor pressure of water at that temperature. Table 2-1 shows how the vapor pressure of water varies as a function of temperature. When the partial pressure of water in a wet gas is equal to its maximum value at the existing temperature, the gas is said to be saturated with water vapor. Relative humidity of a gas is defined as the ratio of the actual partial pressure of water to the vapor pressure at the same temperature, i.e.,

$$\text{relative humidity (\%)} = \frac{100 \times \text{partial pressure of water vapor}}{\text{vapor pressure at same temperature}}$$

If the vapor is in contact with an excess of liquid, then saturation (100% relative humidity) is insured. Thus, in the lung or wet

TABLE 2-1
Vapor Pressure of Water

Temperature (°C)	Vapor Pressure (mm Hg)
20	17.5
21	18.7
22	19.8
23	21.1
24	22.4
25	23.8
26	25.2
27	26.7
28	28.3
29	30.0
30	31.8
31	33.7
32	35.7
33	37.8
34	39.9
35	42.2
36	44.6
37	47.0
38	49.7
39	52.4
40	55.3

spirometer where an ample amount of water is always present, the partial pressure of water vapor equals the vapor pressure of water and is a function of temperature alone. Because water vapor partial pressure is constant at a given temperature, in applying equations (1) and (2) the partial pressure of water vapor must be excluded.

Since temperature and water vapor pressure both influence gas volume, their effects must be considered in any measurement of volume. Thus, if there is a difference in temperature between the measurement apparatus and gas volume of interest, the measured volume must be corrected.

When lung volumes at body temperature are measured with a wet spirometer at room temperature, measured volumes must be corrected to BTPS conditions (body temperature, pressure saturated). Thus, if a wet spirometer volume V_1 is measured at temperature T_1 (°C), barometric pressure B (mm Hg), and water vapor pressure $P_1(H_2O)$, then the volume V(BTPS) is

$$V(BTPS) = \frac{V_1 \times [B - P_1(H_2O)] \times (273 + 37)}{(B - 47) \times (273 + T_1)} \quad (4)$$

where $P_1(H_2O)$ is the vapor pressure of water at temperature T_1. Equation (4) is merely an application of equation (1) when the mass of gas is a constant. The constant value of 273 is used to convert °C to °K.

When the number of gas molecules is of primary interest, volumes are expressed at standard temperature (0°C), standard pressure (760 mm Hg), and dry (STPD). Oxygen consumption, carbon dioxide production, and diffusing capacity are examples where STPD units are used. Similarly, as above, if volume V_1 is measured at temperature T_1, barometric pressure B, and saturated water vapor, then the volume V(STPD) is

$$V(STPD) = \frac{V_1 + [B - P_1(H_2O)] \times (273)}{760 \times (273 + T_1)} \qquad (5)$$

Henry's Law

When a liquid and gas are in equilibrium, the amount of gas in solution is directly proportional to the partial pressure of the gas provided temperature is constant. The following equation describes this behavior:

$$C_g = A\alpha_g P_g$$

where C_g is the gas concentration in solution, α_g is the Bunsen solubility coefficient, P_g is the gas partial pressure, and A is a constant whose value depends on the system of units used. For C_g measured in terms of volume % (ml/100 ml) and α_g given in ml/ml solvent, A = 0.132 for P_g measured in units of mm Hg. The values of α_g in the above units are listed in Table 2-2 for various gases.

TABLE 2-2
Bunsen Solubility Coefficients
[ml (STPD)/ml solvent, P_g = 760 mm Hg, T = 37°C]

Gas	α_g	
	Plasma	Blood*
He	0.0154	0.0149
N_2	0.0117	0.0130
O_2	0.0209	0.0240
CO_2	0.5100	0.4700

*Hematocrit = 0.45.

Applications

DETERMINATION OF THORACIC GAS VOLUME

The compressibility of a gas (dV/dP) under constant temperature conditions is easily obtained by differentiating equation (2), yielding

$$\frac{dV}{dP} = \frac{d}{dP}\left(\frac{\text{constant}}{P}\right)$$

$$= -\frac{\text{constant}}{P^2}$$

$$= -\frac{V}{P} \tag{6}$$

By rearranging the above equation,

$$V = -P\frac{dV}{dP} \tag{7}$$

The above equation is useful, since it provides a means of measuring a gas volume when direct measurements are impossible. Thus it is possible to estimate the volume of a gas at constant temperature if gas pressure and compressibility are measured. This approach has been taken to measure thoracic gas volume (1). To accomplish this, a subject with a noseclip attached is instructed to make several respiratory efforts against a closed mouthpiece following the end of a normal expiration. Mouth pressure and volume changes are measured with a straingage and body plethysmograph, respectively. Since temperature is constant at body temperature (37°C), equation (7) is applicable. The ratio of the change in volume (ΔV) and pressure (ΔP) is used to estimate compressibility. The initial pressure P_1 (atmospheric) minus the vapor pressure of water at body temperature (47 mm Hg) is then multiplied by compressibility to yield thoracic gas volume.

MEASUREMENT OF ALVEOLAR PRESSURE

During breathing, the actions of the respiratory muscles on the chest compress and expand the gas within the alveoli. The resultant alveolar pressure is the force which then drives gas through the airway. Its measurement is necessary to estimate airway resistance and can be accomplished using the following form of equation (6):

$$\Delta P_{alv} = \frac{[B - P_{(H_2O)}] \times \Delta V}{V_L} \tag{8}$$

The Δ indicates a change in conditions from the end of expiration. Since alveolar pressure equals atmospheric pressure at the end of expiration, ΔP_{alv} is the net force that moves air through the airway. The alveolar volume compression or expansion, ΔV is readily measured with a body plethysmograph. Also $P_{(H_2O)}$ is the vapor pressure of water at body temperature, and V_L is the thoracic lung volume, which can be determined as described previously. Although equation (8) is strictly true only for an infinitesimally small change in volume and pressure, total changes in pressure and volume are usually small enough to permit application of (2).

Gas Law Problems

You will need to know the barometric pressure at various altitudes to work the problems. These are given in Table 2-3.

TABLE 2-3
U.S. Standard Atmosphere

Altitude (ft)	Barometric Pressure (mm Hg)	(atm)	Altitude (ft)	Barometric Pressure (mm Hg)	(atm)
0	760	1	27,500	253	0.333
5,000	632	0.832	30,000	226	0.297
10,000	523	0.688	33,700	190	0.250
15,000	429	0.565	38,300	152	0.200
18,000	380	0.500	40,000	141	0.185
20,000	349	0.460	45,000	111	0.146
25,000	282	0.371	63,000	47	0.062

1. If the pressure of O_2 in a cylinder supplying an O_2 tent falls during use from an initial 1800 lb/in.^{2} to 600 lb/in.^{2}, what fraction of the initial supply remains in the cylinder?
2. (a) Calculate the P_{O_2} of dry atmospheric air at sea level. (b) Would this number be any different if the N_2 were replaced volume for volume by helium?
3. Breathing air deficient in O_2 is called simple anoxia; the absolute concentration is what the body "sees," and it may be reduced in either of the following ways: (a) Calculate the P_{O_2} of 10.5% O_2 at sea level. (b) Calculate the P_{O_2} of atmospheric air at 18,000 ft.
4. Breathing air containing CO_2 is called CO_2 inhalation; again, it is the absolute concentration that the body "sees." (a) Calculate the

% CO_2 that must be added to yield a P_{CO_2} of 38 mm Hg at sea level. (b) at 18,000 ft.
5. What is the P_{H_2O} of alveolar air in normal persons (a) at sea level? (b) at 18,000 ft? (c) in a febrile patient with a temperature of 104°F (40°C)?
6. What % of total alveolar pressure is pre-empted by water vapor (a) at sea level? (b) at 33,700 ft? (c) at 63,000 ft? (d) What would happen to tissue water at the latter altitude? (e) Would you expect the anoxia of altitude to be related to the PO_2 of dry atmospheric air or to that of air saturated with water at body temperature? (f) Which has the lower PO_2?
7. A subject's basal O_2 consumption measured in the spirometer (wet, T = 20°C, B = 730 mm Hg) was 0.310 L/min. (a) What is this, properly corrected to STPD? (b) Improperly corrected to BTPS? (c) What is the % error for the latter? This error is large enough to lead to a misdiagnosis of hyperthyroidism in a perfectly normal patient.
8. A subject had a normal vital capacity of 5.0 liters at sea level. When tested again at 20,000 ft altitude, the spirometer volume (wet, 20°C) was 4.3 liters. (a) What is his vital capacity at the higher altitude? (b) Did altitude affect it?
9. (a) Calculate the tracheal P_{O_2} for atmospheric air at sea level. (b) Calculate the % CO_2 required to yield a tracheal P_{CO_2} of 35 mm Hg.
10. (a) Calculate the P_{O_2} of alveolar at sea level containing the normal 14.6% O_2. (b) Calculate the P_{CO_2} of alveolar air at sea level containing the normal 5.62% CO_2. (c) During short exposure to 18,000 ft the alveolar P_{CO_2} falls to about 32 mm Hg. What % CO_2 is this?
11. (a) Calculate the vol % of physically dissolved O_2 in arterial blood in equilibrium with a normal alveolar P_{O_2} of 104 mm Hg. (b) Since the total O_2 content of arterial blood is about 20 vol %, what % must be bound to Hb?
12. (a) Calculate the vol % of physically dissolved CO_2 in arterial blood in equilibrium with a normal alveolar P_{CO_2} of 40 mm Hg. (b) Since the total CO_2 content of arterial blood is about 49 vol %, what % must be bound as $BHCO_3$ and carbamate?
13. (a) At rest, the P_{O_2} of mixed venous blood delivered to the lungs is about 40 mm Hg, whereas the alveolar P_{O_2} is about 104 mm Hg. When the blood reaches the alveoli, will it pick up or give off O_2? (b) At rest, the P_{CO_2} of mixed venous blood is about 47 mm Hg, whereas the alveolar P_{CO_2} is about 40. When the blood reaches the alveoli, will it pick up or give off CO_2?

GAS LAWS AND APPLICATIONS 15

ANSWERS TO GAS LAW PROBLEMS

1. $\frac{600}{1800} = \frac{1}{3}$
2. (a) $760 \times 0.21 = 160$ mm Hg
   (b) No
3. (a) $760 \times 0.105 = 80$ mm Hg
   (b) $380 \times 0.21 = 80$ mm Hg
4. (a) $\frac{38}{760} = 5\%$
   (b) $\frac{38}{380} = 10\%$
5. (a) 47 mm Hg
   (b) 47 mm Hg
   (c) 55 mm Hg
6. (a) $\frac{47}{760} = 6.2\%$
   (b) $\frac{47}{190} = 24.8\%$
   (c) $\frac{47}{47} = 100\%$
   (d) Boil
   (e) Saturated
   (f) Saturated
7. (a) $\dfrac{273}{293} \times \dfrac{730-18}{760} \times 0.310 = 0.271$ L/min (STPD)
   (b) $\dfrac{310}{293} \times \dfrac{730-18}{730-47} \times 0.310 = 0.342$ L/min (BTPS)
   (c) $\dfrac{0.342 - 0.271}{0.271} = 26\%$ error (2 CV's)
8. (a) $\dfrac{310}{293} \times \dfrac{349-18}{349-47} \times 4.3 = 5.0$ L (BTPS)
   (b) No—it should not.
9. (a) $(760 - 47)0.21 = 150$ mm Hg
   (b) $35/(760 - 47) = 5\%$ (dry)
10. (a) $(760 - 47)0.146 = 104$ mm Hg
    (b) $(760 - 47)0.0562 = 40$ mm Hg
    (c) $32/(380 - 47) = 9.6\%$ (dry)
11. (a) $0.132 \times 0.024 \times 104 = 0.33$ vol % (STPD)
    (b) $\dfrac{20 - 0.33}{20} = 98\%$
12. (a) $0.132 \times 0.47 \times 40 = 2.6$ vol %(STPD)
    (b) $\dfrac{49 - 2.6}{49} = 95\%$
13. (a) Pick up O_2
    (b) Give off CO_2

References

1. DuBois, A. B., S. Y. Botelho, G. N. Bedell, R. Marshall, and J. H. Comroe, Jr. Rapid plethysmographic method for measuring thoracic gas volume:

Comparison with nitrogen washout method for measuring functional residual capacity in normal subjects. *J. Clin. Invest.* **35**: 322–326, 1956.

2. DuBois, A. B., S. Y. Botelho, and J. H. Comroe, Jr. New methods for measuring airway resistance in man using body plethysmographs: Values in normal subjects and patients with respiratory disease. *J. Clin. Invest.* **35**: 327–335, 1956.

CHAPTER 3

The Ventilatory Apparatus

THE VENTILATORY APPARATUS has the task of producing an alternating bulk flow of gas between the external atmosphere and the lung alveoli. It consists of the respiratory muscles, which furnish the energy, and the lung-thorax pump, which these muscles alternately expand in inspiration and release for passive recoil or actively compress in expiration. Since this component operates as a purely mechanical pump, it is convenient to consider in sequence its geometrics (i.e., static size characteristics), its kinematics (i.e., its geometrics as they change in time), and its dynamics (i.e., the forces involved in its motion).

Geometrics

The total lung capacity is divided into four primary lung volumes, which are, in turn, recombined in various ways to define three special lung capacities (Figure 3-1). For purposes of description, it is also convenient to define the four chest "positions" as shown in the figure. All of the primary lung volumes except the residual volume can be measured by direct spirometry, i.e., by utilizing a device (spirometer) that collects gas over water in a calibrated, counterbalanced bell (Figure 3-2). What the spirometer measures is a volume of wet gas at spirometer temperature and pressure. What we really want to know is the volume occupied by this gas when it is in the lung at body

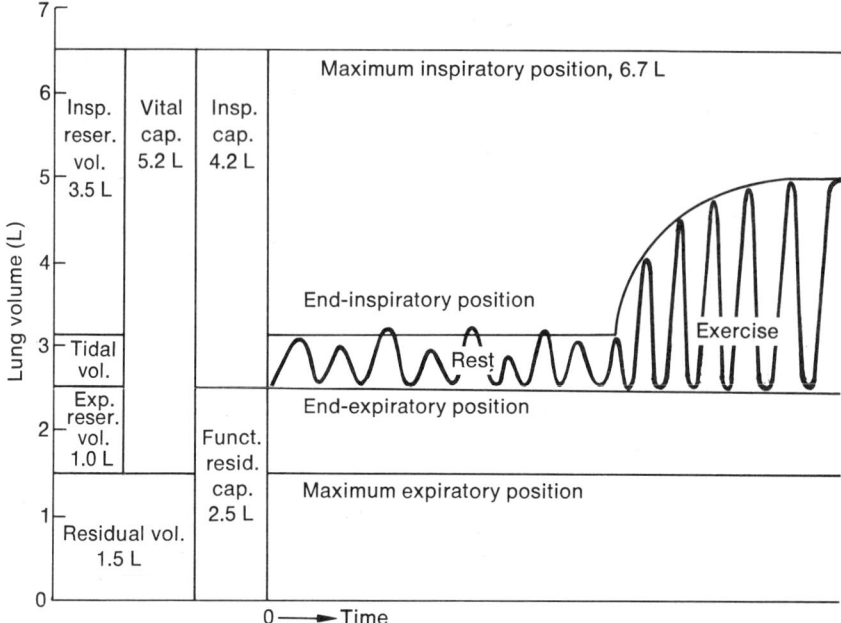

FIGURE 3-1. Static lung volumes. Values correspond to a healthy, young adult male.

temperature and pressure. Hence these spirometer volumes are always corrected to BTPS.

Figure 3-1 should be self-explanatory; we shall not attempt to give verbal definitions for all of these quantities. We note, however, that the tidal volume is the volume of a single breath, that its maximum possible value is the vital capacity, and that since the residual volume remains behind after a maximum expiration, it cannot be collected in a spirometer for direct measurement. It can be measured by dilution techniques or by the body plethysmograph. The latter can measure FRC directly, and since expiratory reserve volume can be measured easily by direct spirometry, residual volume can be obtained by difference. Finally, we note that the FRC provides a "buffer" against wide swings in the composition of alveolar gas during the respiratory cycle.

Kinematics

The spirometer record (*spirogram*) in Figure 3-1 is a kinematic description of the changes in lung volume with time during the

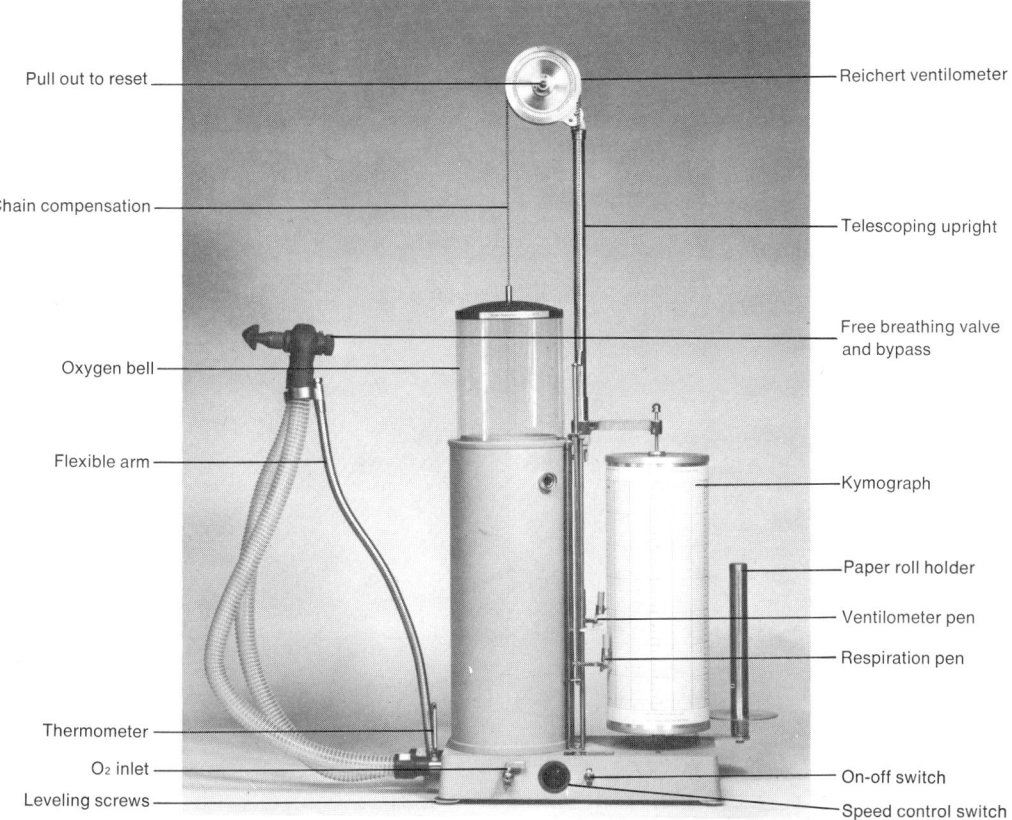

FIGURE 3-2. Collins 9-liter respirometer. (Courtesy of Warren E. Collins, Inc., Braintree, Mass.)

respiratory cycle. If we temporarily ignore the cyclic nature of the pump, we can define pulmonary ventilation, $\dot{V}$, as the volume of air expired (or inspired) in 1 min. We can calculate it from the spirogram in Figure 3-1 by adding the tidal volumes over 1 min, or we could simply collect only expired air in a spirometer for 1 min. Normal resting $\dot{V}$ is about 7 L/min and it may rise to 120 L/min in severe exercise. Normal resting breathing is called *eupnea*, any increase above eupnea is called *hyperpnea*, and if breathing stops, we have *apnea*. If we ask a normal subject to breathe "as hard as he can" during 15 to 20 sec and convert this to its equivalent $\dot{V}$, we get values around 170 L/min. We call this the *ventilation capacity*, $\dot{V}C$, and it exceeds the levels reached during exercise. An obvious derived quantity is the *ventilatory reserve*, $\dot{V}R$, defined somewhat awkwardly in words as the % of the ventilation capacity still available at a given level of ventilation, or more compactly in symbols as:

$$\dot{V}R = 100\left(\frac{\dot{V}C - \dot{V}}{\dot{V}C}\right)$$

Now turning our attention to the cycle itself, we note that $\dot{V}$ is really the product of tidal volume, V_T, and frequency, f. If we differentiate the spirogram in Figure 3-1 with respect to time, we shall obtain a corresponding record of volume flow rate, $\dot{V}(t)$, as a function of time. This is called a *pneumotachogram* and is shown along with the corresponding spirogram in Figure 3-3. The pneumotachogram can also

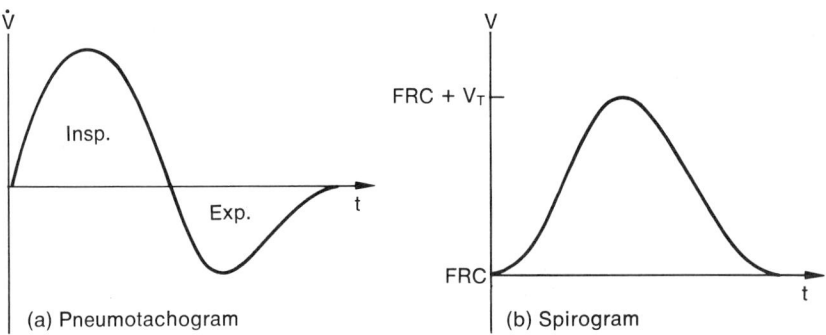

FIGURE 3-3. Relationship between pneumotachogram (airflow) and spirogram (volume). The pattern corresponds to eupnea.

be obtained directly by having the subject breathe through a suitable flowmeter (*pneumotachograph*, PTG). The human pneumotachogram in eupnea, although it may superficially resemble a sine wave, is actually quite asymmetrical. Thus the expiratory phase is about 20% longer in duration than the inspiratory phase, and the peak inspiratory flow rate is about 10% higher than peak expiratory flow. It is convenient to remember that mean pulmonary ventilation, $\dot{V}$, is about one third of the peak inspiratory flow rate. In the normal hyperpnea of exercise, both frequency and tidal volume increase, but in disease (e.g., pneumonia), the frequency may increase greatly while tidal volume falls. Such rapid shallow breathing is called *tachypnea*.

Dynamics

THE LUMPED LUNG-THORAX MODEL

In 1915, the Swiss physiologist Fritz Rohrer (*15*) published a classic study of respiratory mechanics that has provided the basis for most

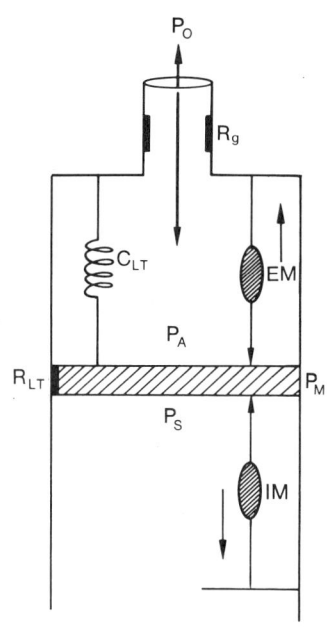

FIGURE 3-4. Mechanical analog of the ventilatory apparatus.

of the work in this area since that time. It is most convenient to describe the dynamics of the ventilatory apparatus in terms of the equivalent piston pump shown in Figure 3-4. Its essential components are the inspiratory and expiratory muscles that provide the energy to drive the piston, and the elastic and resistive elements against which they must work. To begin with, we consider the lungs and the thorax as a lumped structure characterized by a single equivalent elastic element and a single equivalent resistive element. We recall that an elastic element is a static component that develops a stress (force) dependent upon its position (strain), whereas a resistive element is a dynamic component that develops a force dependent on rate of change of position, i.e., velocity. When the inspiratory muscles apply a force to expand the lung-thorax (i.e., pull the piston down in Figure 3-4), the elastic tissues act as a spring and thus oppose the motion. In addition, the tissues have a sort of internal viscosity (or resistance) that also opposes the motion. Finally, the flow of gas through the tracheobronchial tree is opposed by resistive forces generated by gas viscosity.

The "equation of motion" is simply a statement of the physical principle that the driving force must be equal to the sum of the opposing forces at every instant. In respiratory mechanics we are accustomed to dealing with pressures and volumes rather than forces and distances, and we write our equations in this form. It is also customary to use volume compliance (i.e., $\Delta V/\Delta P$) rather than volume elastance (i.e., $\Delta P/\Delta V$) to represent the elastic properties. We also note that the unstressed position (volume) of C_{LT} is FRC. Finally, inertial forces are usually small enough to be neglected. We are thus led to the following equation of motion for the respiratory pump:

$$\text{sum of opposing pressures} = \text{driving pressure}$$

$$\text{resistive pressure} + \text{elastic pressure} = \text{driving pressure}$$

$$P_R + P_E = P_M$$

$$(R_{LT} + R_g)\dot{V} + \frac{1}{C_{LT}}V = P_M$$

where

V = (lung-thorax volume—FRC), liters,
$\dot{V}$ = rate of change of lung-thorax volume ≡ volume flow rate, 1/min,
P_O = oral pressure (normally, 0 ≡ atmospheric),
P_S = body surface pressure (normally, 0 ≡ atmospheric),
P_M = muscle driving pressure, cm H_2O,
C_{LT} = compliance of lungs-thorax, $\Delta V/\Delta P_E$, l/cm H_2O,
R_{LT} = viscous resistance of lungs-thorax, $\Delta P_{RLT}/\Delta \dot{V}$, and
R_g = viscous resistance of gas, $\Delta P_{R_g}/\Delta \dot{V}$.

An equivalent electrical circuit is given in Figure 3-5. The equation, as written, implicitly assumes that the system is linear; i.e., R_{LT}, R_g, and C_{LT} are all constant and independent of $\dot{V}$ and/or V. We shall see later how far this assumption can be pushed.

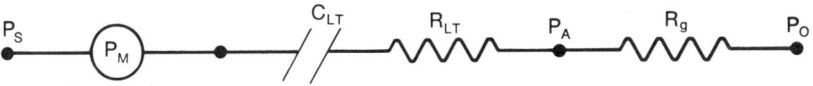

FIGURE 3-5.   Electrical analog of the ventilatory apparatus.

What does such an equation of motion do for us? It gives us a compact dynamic description of the operation of the respiratory pump in the sense that if we know the muscular driving function $[P_M(t)]$ and the passive elastic and resistive properties of the pump (C_{LT}, R_{LT}, R_g), then the solution of the equation will tell us how V and $\dot{V}$ will vary with time as the pump operates. This leads naturally to the question, how do we determine $P_M(t)$, C_{LT}, R_{LT}, and R_g? Let us begin with the easiest problem, i.e., the measurement of C_{LT}.

ELASTIC PROPERTIES. Although the actual deformation of the lung-thorax tissue during the respiratory cycle is hardly a volume strain, description of pump dynamics (in contrast to a rigorous description of tissue elasticity) need only be concerned with the static relationship between the pressure drop across the lung-thorax and lung volume. This is relatively easily measured by having a subject relax his muscles while known pressures are applied at the mouth and the resultant changes in lung volume determined. A plot of lung volume vs. oral pressure determined in this way is called a *relaxation pressure-volume curve*; an example for a normal man is shown in Figure 3-6.

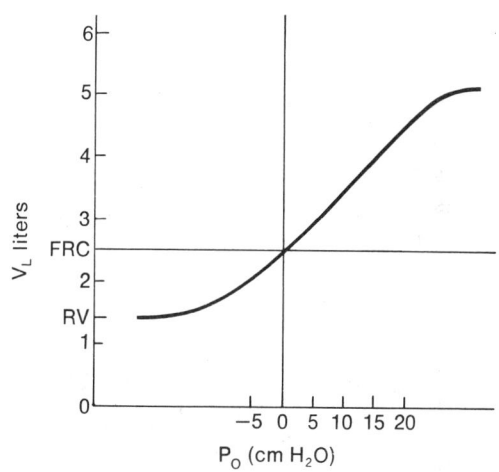

FIGURE 3-6. Relaxation pressure-volume curve for lung-thorax combination.

We note that the curve is nonlinear, having a sigmoid shape. Fortunately, however, the usual range of operation is included between V = 2 liters and V = 4 liters, and here a linear approximation with a constant slope, $\Delta V/\Delta P = 0.1$ liter/cm $H_2O \equiv C_{LT}$ is an adequate description of the compliance. We note also that the unstressed volume of the lung-thorax ($V_0 \equiv V$ at $P_0 = 0$) is the FRC, normally about 2.5 liters.

This curve is due partly to the elastic properties of the lung tissue, partly to the elastic properties of the thorax, and partly to surface tension effects at the alveolar liquid-gas interface. We shall look at these separately later, and simply note here that in disease, either the slope, C_{LT}, or the unstressed volume, FRC, or both, may change. Thus FRC is increased in both senile and chronic obstructive emphysema, but in the former C_{LT} is much reduced, whereas in the latter, it is somewhat increased.

Having described the measurement of C_{LT}, let us now turn to the determination of R_g and R_{LT}.

RESISTIVE PROPERTIES. The resistive properties of our ventilatory pump are really operationally defined by a plot of the volume flow rate of gas, $\dot{V}(t)$, as a function of the pressure drop producing it, P_R. The former, except for usually negligible gas compression effects, is equal to the rate of change of lung volume and can easily be measured directly from a pneumotachogram (PTG) or by differentiation of a spirogram (SPG). But how do we measure P_R?

We recall from our equation of motion that our total driving pressure during normal breathing, $P_M(t)$, is equal at every instant to the sum of two pressures, $P_E = (1/C_{LT})V$, and $P_R = (R_g + R_{LT})\dot{V}$. To measure C_{LT}, we set $P_M = 0$ (relaxed muscles), and substituted a known oral driving pressure, P_O, which we made equal to P_E by measuring V under static conditions, i.e., when $\dot{V} = 0 = P_R$. An analogous "trick" to measure $(R_g + R_{LT})$ would be to again set $P_M = 0$, substitute a known oral driving pressure, P_O, and make it equal to P_R by measuring $\dot{V}$ only when V is at FRC where $P_E = 0$. This is obviously impractical. What we actually do is to set $P_M = 0$ (relaxed muscles), substitute a known periodic driving pressure at the mouth, $P_O(t)$, or lung-thorax surface, $P_S(t)$ (i.e., we use artificial respiration) and record $P_O(t)$, $\dot{V}(t)$, and $V(t)$ continuously. We know that at every instant, $P_O(t) = P_E(t) + P_R(t)$. We also know that $P_E(t) = (1/C_{LT})V(t)$, so that if we determine C_{LT} as already described, we can calculate $P_R(t) = P_O(t) - (1/C_{LT})V(t)$. Then for every t, we have corresponding values of P_R and $\dot{V}$, and we can plot the pressure-flow curve that defines the resistive properties of our system. When we do this, we get the curve shown in Figure 3-7.

We note first that this curve expresses total resistive forces, $R = (R_g + R_{LT})$, and second that it is nonlinear. If we define R as the reciprocal of the slope of this curve, i.e., $\Delta P_R/\Delta \dot{V}$, it is clear that R is not a constant but increases with increasing $\dot{V}$. This nonlinearity is probably mainly due to turbulent gas flow that occurs locally in the larynx even in eupnea and becomes increasingly widespread with increasing hyperpnea (*vide infra*). However, for flows up to moderate hyperpnea, we can use a linear approximation with a slope, $R = 0.045$ cm $H_2O/L/min$. If we use these linearized values for both C_{LT} and R, then it is clear from the equation of motion that V should fall exponentially during a passive expiration with a time constant, $T \equiv RC_{LT} = 0.045 \times 0.1 = 0.0045$ min or 0.27 sec.

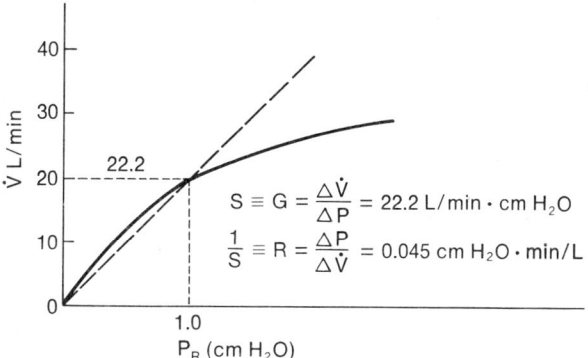

FIGURE 3-7. Total respiratory system pressure-flow curve.

How can we separate R into its two components, R_{LT} and R_g? To do this, we should have to divide the total resistive drop from mouth to body surface, P_R, into two series components, ΔP_{R_g} from mouth to alveolar space, and $\Delta P_{R_{LT}}$ from alveolar space to body surface. To do this, we need to be able to measure the pressure in the alveolar space, P_A (Figures 3-4 and 3-5). Because the alveoli are so small, it is not practical to do this directly by placing a catheter there. An early indirect method consisted of momentarily closing the airway during the respiratory cycle and measuring the pressure proximal to the obstruction. It was assumed that since there was now no flow, this pressure would equal the alveolar pressure just prior to the block. It has since been found that this is a dangerous assumption, primarily because of the influence of inertial forces. Alveolar pressures are now usually measured by the body plethysmograph (see p. 12). This is a closed rigid chamber in which the subject can sit comfortably and breathe with his airway open either to the plethysmograph or to the external environment. Volume changes, ΔV, associated with the respiratory cycle can be determined from plethysmograph pressure changes, ΔP_P, and these represent compressional effects only (if the airway is closed or is open to the plethysmograph) or compressional plus bulk flow effects (if the airway is open to the outside). To measure the P_A associated with a particular $\dot{V}$, $\dot{V}$ and ΔV are first measured during rapid shallow rebreathing through a PTG open to the plethysmograph. The airway is then blocked and mouth pressure, P_O, and ΔV are measured while the subject continues his breathing efforts against the closed airway. It is assumed that $P_O = P_A$ during these purely compressional changes with no air flow at the mouth. Since changes in P_A always depend on compressional effects, it is further assumed that the P_A measured with airway closed at any given ΔV is also the P_A at

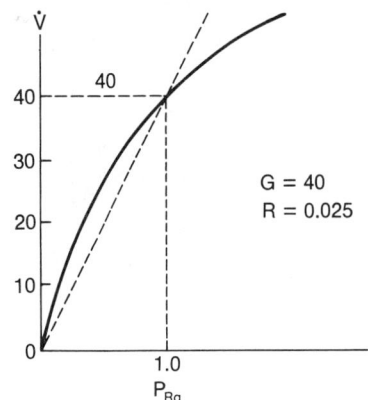

FIGURE 3-8. Gas pressure-flow curve.

the same ΔV with airway open. Hence corresponding values for P_A and $\dot{V}$ can be obtained. Plotting these values yields a curve very similar in shape to that of Figure 3-7, as shown in Figure 3-8. If we use a linear approximation for $\Delta P/\Delta \dot{V}$ for eupnea to moderate hyperpnea, we get $R_g = 0.025 \text{ cmH}_2\text{O/L/min}$, or about 56% of $(R_g + R_{LT})$. By difference, $R_{LT} = 0.020$.

Since Figure 3-8 represents only airway resistance to bulk gas flow, let us briefly examine the effects of flow pattern on airflow resistance in an effort to account for its shape. Flow may be purely laminar, purely turbulent, or some combination of the two. In purely laminar flow, the fluid moves as if it were composed of concentric stream tubes that slide one inside the other. The axial tube moves with maximum velocity; the outermost tube moves not at all; and the velocities of those in between increase parabolically from zero at the wall to a maximum at the axis (*parabolic velocity profile*, Figure 3-9). The opposing force in this sort of flow is generated by the viscous friction between sliding stream tubes, and the fluid property that contributes to it is the dynamic viscosity, μ, defined as the ratio of shear stress to rate of shear

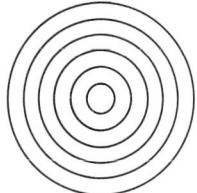 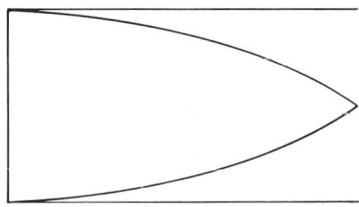

FIGURE 3-9. Parabolic velocity profile.

strain whose units are therefore

$$\frac{\text{dynes}}{\text{cm}^2} \Big/ \frac{\text{cm/sec}}{\text{cm}} = \frac{\text{dyne sec}}{\text{cm}^2} = \frac{\text{g}}{\text{cm sec}} \equiv \text{poise}$$

The term *poise* comes, of course, from the name of the French physician (not physicist or engineer) who defined the factors relating pressure drop to flow rate in laminar flow through cylindrical tubes in 1836, Poiseuille. Poiseuille's law is

$$\dot{V} = P_R \left(\frac{\pi r^4}{8 \ell \mu} \right)$$

where r = tube radius,
ℓ = tube length, and
μ = the dynamic viscosity defined above.

It is clear that for a fluid in a given tube, $\dot{V}$ is directly proportional to P_R with proportionality constant $\pi r^4 / 8 \ell \mu \equiv 1/R$, and is thus a linear function of P_R. The dynamic viscosity of air is 180 μ poise and of helium 203 μ poise at 37°C. Laminar flow is literally "silent" and generates neither breath sounds nor cardiovascular sounds.

Turbulent flow is characterized by irregular flow paths at various angles to the main axis of flow. It may be locally generated by geometric irregularities (e.g., rough walls, constriction, dilatation, branching) but becomes general at high velocities. The *critical velocity* for general turbulence can be obtained from the *Reynolds number*, a dimensionless ratio of inertial to viscous forces:

$$N_R = \frac{\rho \bar{v} D}{\mu}$$

where $N_R \equiv$ Reynolds number,
ρ = fluid density,
μ = fluid viscosity,
$\bar{v}$ = mean linear velocity, and
D = tube diameter.

If $N_R > 2000$, general turbulence usually develops, so the critical velocity is

$$\bar{v}_c = \frac{2000}{D} \left(\frac{\mu}{\rho} \right).$$

The ratio of viscosity to density, μ/ρ, is called the kinematic viscosity, ν (unit = stoke).

In turbulent flow, the relationship between $\dot{V}$ and P_R is no longer linear:

$$\dot{V} = \left(\frac{1}{R_T}\right) P_R^{1/2}$$

where the *turbulent resistance* is a function of tube geometry and fluid density.

Because He mixtures are often substituted for air in efforts to lower airway resistance in disease, it is instructive to ask under what conditions this is likely to be successful. Table 3-1 lists μ, ρ, and ν for He and for air:

TABLE 3-1

	μ (poise × 10^6)	ρ g/L	ν (stokes × 10^6)
air	180	1.12	161
He	203	0.156	1295
He/air	1.13	0.14	8.04

It is clear from Table 3-1 that substitution of He for N_2 can reduce resistance either by converting turbulent flow to laminar flow (because of high ν) or by reducing resistance to turbulent flow (because of low ρ). However, if the flow is laminar for air, substitution of He will actually increase the resistance (because of higher μ).

DETERMINATION OF $P_M(t)$. Returning to our equation of motion, we have now successfully measured C_{LT}, R_{LT}, and R_g. If we now knew $P_M(t)$, solution of our equation would predict the behavior of $V(t)$ and $\dot{V}(t)$ during the respiratory cycle. Unfortunately, it turns out that there is no direct way to measure $P_M(t)$ and we actually end up using the equation of motion to obtain it by solving the so-called converse problem, i.e., given C_{LT}, R_{LTg}, $V(t)$, and $\dot{V}(t)$ during normal breathing, determine $P_M(t)$. It is clear that

$$R_{LTg}\dot{V}(t) + \frac{1}{C_{LT}}V(t) = P_M(t)$$

and $P_M(t)$ so obtained during eupnea is plotted along with $\dot{V}(t)$ and $V(t)$

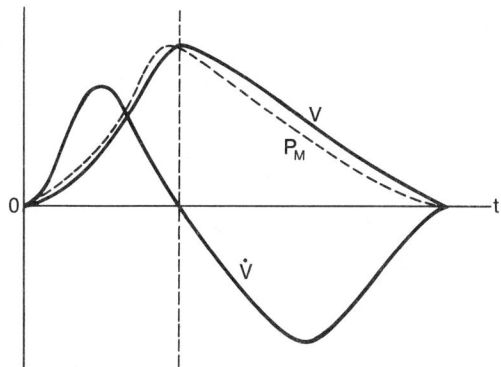

FIGURE 3-10. Relationship between muscle driving pressure (P_M), airflow ($\dot{V}$), and volume (V) in eupnea.

in Figure 3-10. We note that $P_M(t)$ is similar in shape to V(t) but leads it slightly, indicating the importance of the compliance element. We note also that $P_M(t)$ does not suddenly drop to zero at the end of inspiration but instead gradually decreases throughout the entire expiratory phase. This means that eupneic expiration is actually opposed by the continued activity of the inspiratory muscles, the expiratory muscles remaining inactive. During hyperpnea, both sets of muscles become active, and $P_M(t)$ now resembles $\dot{V}(t)$, indicating the increased importance of the resistance factor at high flow rates. It is of interest also that $\dot{V}(t)$ assumes a nearly rectangular shape, which turns out to be the flow pattern that minimizes respiratory work for a given alveolar ventilation. Having introduced the notion of respiratory work, let us take a closer look at what it is and how it is measured.

RESPIRATORY WORK. In driving the respiratory cycle, the respiratory muscles do mechanical work on the lung-thorax pump, definable as $\int P\,dV$. This total work and its components can be obtained from a plot of P_M vs. volume for a complete respiratory cycle. However, since P_M cannot be measured directly during spontaneous breathing, we measure $(P_O - P_S)$ during "normally patterned" artificial respiration with the muscles relaxed, or we calculate P_M indirectly during spontaneous breathing as described above.

A typical PV plot for a eupneic respiratory cycle in man is shown in Figure 3-11. The total work during inspiration is given by the area AICBA, and a typical value is 2910 g cm. This total is made up of two components, elastic work (area ACBA = 2350 g cm), which is stored as potential energy in the distended chest, and resistive work (area AICA = 560 g cm), which is lost as heat. During expiration, the

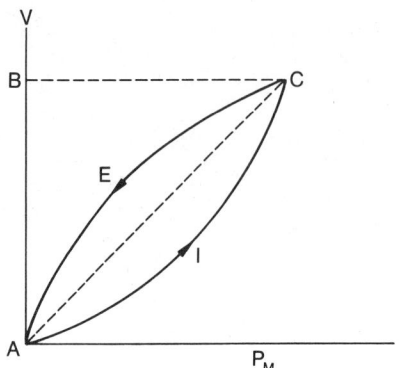

FIGURE 3-11. Dynamic pressure-volume changes during normal breathing.

2350 g cm of potential energy stored during inspiration is used to overcome resistive forces (area ACEA = 440 g cm) and to stretch the inspiratory muscles (area AECBA = 1910 g cm) which, as noted above, actively oppose expiration. This latter component is called "negative work."

The total "useful work" during the eupneic cycle is the 2910 g cm done by the inspiratory muscles during inspiration. If f = 10 cmp, then the "useful power" is 29,100 g cm/min (6.81 × 10^{-4} kg cal/min, 6.37 × 10^{-5} H.P., 0.05 watt!). If the muscles were 100% efficient, this would be equivalent to an oxygen consumption of about 1.4 ml/min, or only about 0.5% of the resting $\dot{V}_{O_2}$ of 275 ml/min.

SEPARATION OF LUNG AND THORAX DYNAMICS

THE EXTENDED MODEL. The model used thus far (Figure 3-4) lumped together the mechanical properties of the lung and thorax, which could thus be described in terms of the parameters, C_{LT} and R_{LT}. We now wish to separate these two structures and to define corresponding parameters for each. To do this, we use the extended models in Figures 3-12 and 3-13. The piston is now split into two components, the lung above and the thorax below. The two are separated by a potential space, the pleural space, which contains a small quantity of pleural fluid serving to lubricate the apposed visceral and parietal pleural surfaces. The pressure in this potential space can be measured as described below and is called pleural pressure, P_p. The lung and the thorax now each have their own respective compliance (spring), C_L and C_T, and resistance, R_L and R_T. At FRC, the total system is in elastic equilibrium with the lung compliance stretched

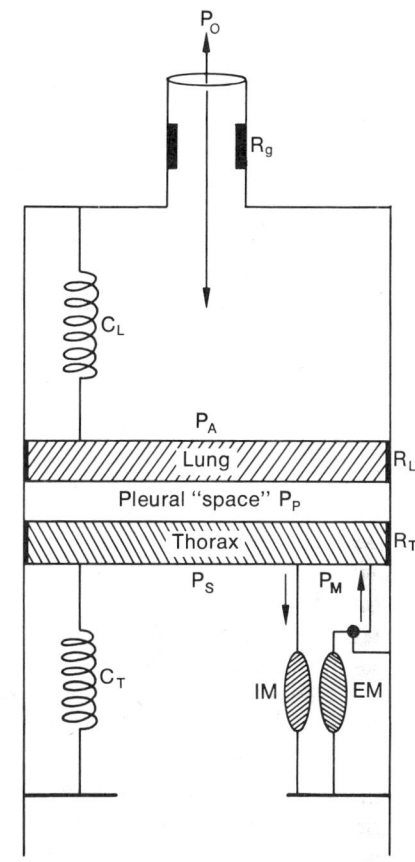

FIGURE 3-12. Mechanical analog of the ventilatory apparatus with separate lung and thoracic components.

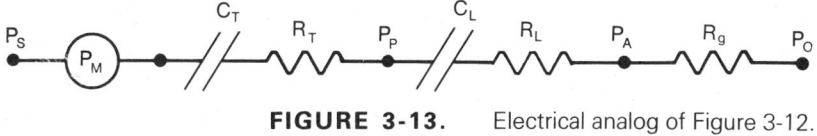

FIGURE 3-13. Electrical analog of Figure 3-12.

beyond its unstressed volume and the thoracic compliance compressed below its unstressed volume.

It should be clear in a qualitative sense that the pressure distending the lung is the transpulmonary pressure ($P_A - P_P$), and the pressure compressing the thorax is the transthoracic pressure ($P_S - P_P$). Since, under static conditions (no flow), $P_A = P_O = P_S = 0$, it is clear that this elastic equilibrium must be manifested by a negative pleural pressure. Finally, it follows that if the pleural space were now freely opened to the atmosphere, thus reducing both transpulmonary and transthoracic pressures to zero (pneumothorax), the lungs would collapse and the thorax would expand to their respective unstressed volumes.

When the diaphragm (IM) contracts during inspiration, the thoracic component of the piston is directly pulled down. Since the lung is directly coupled to the thorax by the pleural space, it follows, and its increasing distention is reflected by an increasingly negative pleural pressure. The increase in lung volume so produced reduces the alveolar pressure, P_A (Boyle's law), and thus sets up the gradient, $P_O - P_A$, which produces inspiratory gas flow. When the diaphragm relaxes, the elastic potential energy stored in the lung returns the system to its starting point in a passive expiration.

With this qualitative introduction, let us look more closely at pulmonary elasticity.

PULMONARY ELASTICITY. Since the lungs and thorax are separated by the pleural space, the measurement of pleural pressure permits a separation of their mechanical properties. Pleural pressure can be measured by a needle placed directly through the chest wall into the pleural space but is more conveniently estimated from measurements of intraesophageal pressure with a balloon catheter. At low balloon volumes ($\approx$0.2 ml air), pressure in the lower part of the esophagus equals pleural pressure at lung volumes above 20% of vital capacity (11). Figure 3-14 shows the static inflation-deflation curve of the lungs of a normal subject as a function of transpulmonary (oral-esophageal of $P_O - P_P$) pressure. The inflation and deflation curves usually differ, and it is customary to choose the deflation curve as the best index of lung recoil, since it is argued that during expiration the maximum number of airways and air spaces are open at a given volume (16). The static deflation pressure-volume curve of the lungs changes due to aging (16) and disease (2).

It is instructive to plot the static pressure-volume curve for the lung on the same pressure-volume diagram used previously to show the "relaxation pressure-volume curve" for the lung-thorax combination (p. 23 and Figure 3-6). This has been done in Figure 3-15. Note that the pressure on the abscissa represents the appropriate distending (+) or compressing (−) force, $P_O - P_S$ or simply P_O for the LT combination and $P_O - P_P$ for the lung, with the pressure at the respective unstressed volumes being zero. Since, as we have noted previously, the combined LT curve represents the sum of its individual L and T components, we can derive the isolated thorax elastic characteristic by substracting the transpulmonary pressure from P_O at corresponding volumes.

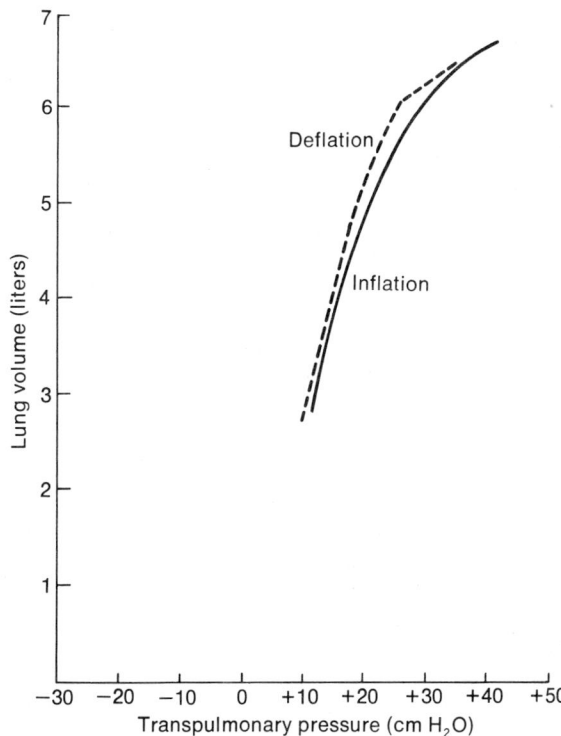

FIGURE 3-14. Inflation-deflation curves of lungs. Volumes are measured from residual volume.

The curve so obtained is also plotted in Figure 3-15. Note that $P_O - (P_O - P_P) = P_P$ so that the transthoracic pressure is simply the pleural pressure with $P_S = 0$.

The reader should become thoroughly familiar with this diagram, understand the relevant pressures and their interrelations, and be able to describe the effects of a pneumothorax in relation to these elastic characteristics.

The elastic behavior of the lung shown in Figure 3-15 is partly due to the elastic properties of lung tissue itself and partly to surface tension effects associated with the normal air-liquid interface at the alveolar surface. This can be most easily demonstrated by comparing deflation pressure-volume curves for animal lungs filled with air with those for lungs filled with saline solution (Figure 3-16). In the latter case, the air-liquid interface is abolished and thus the pure tissue elastic characteristic revealed. The difference between the two curves is due to surface tension effects.

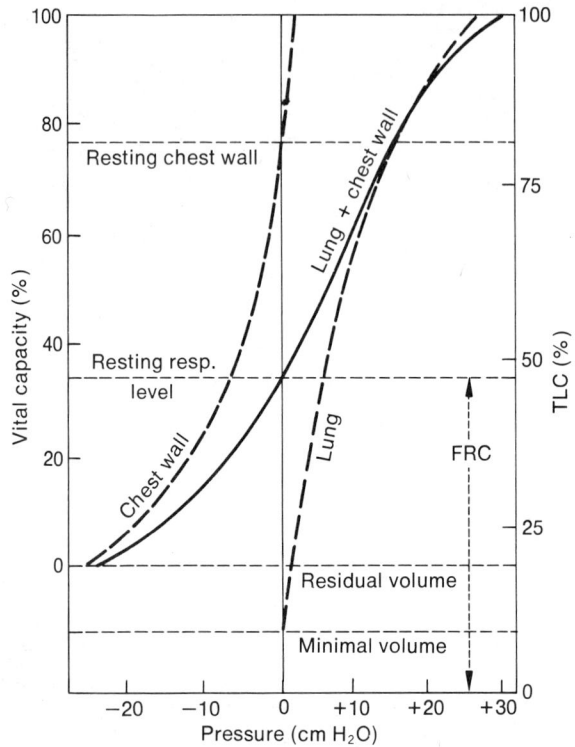

FIGURE 3-15. Relaxation pressure-volume curve for lung-thorax combination and its components. (From J. B. West. *Respiratory Physiology*. Baltimore: The Williams & Wilkins Company, © 1974.)

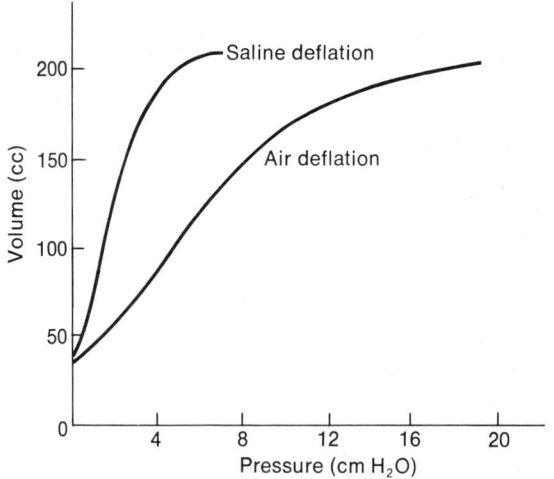

FIGURE 3-16. Comparison of saline and air pressure volume curves. [Data of Radford (6).]

SURFACE TENSION AND SURFACTANT. The consideration of surface tension effects on the elastic properties of the lung provides an excellent example of how theoretical concepts can lead to a very important material discovery. Thus, if we consider an alveolus to be a closed thin-walled sphere, Laplace's law defines the relationship between transmural pressure, P, circumferential wall tension, T, and sphere radius, r, that must hold at equilibrium:

$$P = \frac{2T}{r}$$

Now r for a cat alveolus is about 67 μm and, since P varies between 0 and about 4 cm H_2O during a eupneic respiratory cycle, T by the above formula should vary between 0 and 13 dynes/cm. But if T were completely determined by the surface tension of water at the air-alveolar interface, it ought to have a constant value, independent of r, of some 70 dynes/cm; i.e., the surface tension of pure water is independent of surface area. If T were indeed constant at all values of r, then, if P were reduced, the alveolus should collapse completely. Moreover, if two alveoli of different radii were connected as shown in Figure 3-17, the Laplace relation implies that $P_1 > P_2$ so that when the

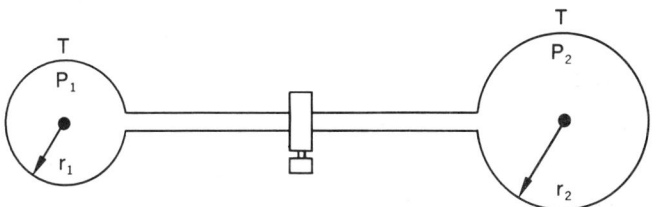

FIGURE 3-17. Model demonstrating instability for constant T.

clamp is released the smaller alveolus would empty into the larger one and thus collapse. Thus pure surface tension effects imply a "negative compliance" and alveolar instability and collapse. Since, in general, alveoli are stable and do not collapse, we seem to have a paradox here that must be resolved.

Over the past 50 years or so, many ingenious solutions were offered to explain this discrepancy [von Neergaard (12), Radford (14), Brown et al. (4)]. This work culminated in the search for, and discovery of, a surface active agent or surfactant that is normally present at the alveolar surface. This substance is a lipoprotein rich in lecithin (dipalmitoyl lecithin) that is probably secreted by the alveolar cells. Its presence not only reduces the alveolar surface tension to about

50 dynes/cm at normal lung volumes but, even more important, it makes T directly dependent on alveolar surface area. Thus T falls to as low as 5 dynes/cm at small lung volumes and general alveolar stability is achieved. Even so, however, stability is not perfect and periodic deep breaths or sighs, which normally occur reflexly, are required to reinflate collapsed units.

Apparently, this pulmonary surfactant only begins to be produced in the fetus near term. Its lack may cause the so-called respiratory distress syndrome or hyaline membrane disease in the newborn.

FREQUENCY DEPENDENCE OF PULMONARY RESISTANCE AND COMPLIANCE. The measurement of pleural pressure permits the determination of the static pressure-volume curve of the lungs as described above. The slope of this curve ($\Delta V/\Delta P$) at a particular lung volume is defined as the static compliance of the lungs. It is also possible to estimate a pulmonary compliance and even resistance while breathing at any frequency if total air flow and transpulmonary pressure are measured simultaneously. Compliance is estimated by taking the ratio of the change in lung volume (ΔV_L) and the change in transpulmonary pressure (ΔP_{TP}) at zero airflow conditions. Since this procedure can be applied when breathing at various frequencies, compliance estimated in this way is called dynamic compliance (C_{dyn}):

$$C_{dyn} = \frac{\Delta V_L}{\Delta P_{TP}}\bigg|_{\dot{V}_L=0}$$

In a similar way, dynamic resistance (R_{dyn}) can be estimated by taking the ratio of the change in transpulmonary pressure (ΔP_{TP}) and the change in total airflow ($\Delta \dot{V}_L$) at a certain level of lung volume (V_L):

$$R_{dyn} = \frac{\Delta P_{TP}}{\Delta \dot{V}_L}\bigg|_{V_L=constant}$$

According to the theory developed by Otis and colleagues (13) uneven ventilation of the lungs is manifested by a decrease in C_{dyn} and R_{dyn} with increasing frequency. This phenomenon is due to time constant (product of compliance and resistance) imbalance between parallel lung units. The mechanical and electrical analogs of two pulmonary pathways are shown in Figure 3-18. The equations developed by Otis et al. for such a model are

$$C_{dyn} = \frac{\omega^2(T_2C_1 + T_1C_2)^2 + (C_1 + C_2)^2}{\omega^2(T_1^2C_2 + T_2^2C_2) + (C_1 + C_2)^2},$$

$$R_{dyn} = \frac{\omega^2 T_1 T_2(T_2C_1 + T_1C_2) + (T_1C_1 + T_2C_2)}{\omega^2(T_2C_1 + T_1C_2)^2 + (C_1 + C_2)^2}$$

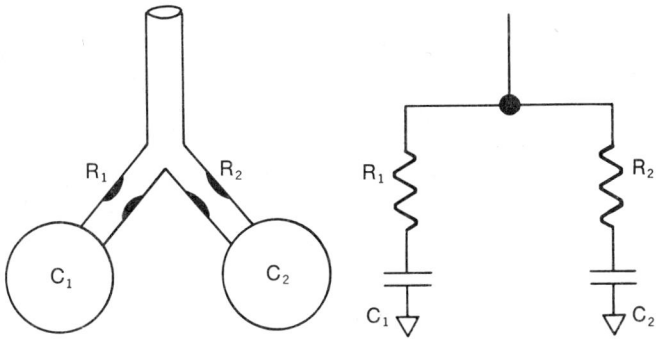

FIGURE 3-18. Mechanical and electrical analogs of two pulmonary pathways.

where $\omega = 2\pi f$ (f = frequency), $T_1 = R_1C_1$, and $T_2 = R_2C_2$. If $T_1 = T_2$, the above equations would reduce to $C_{dyn} = C_1 + C_2$ and $R_{dyn} = R_1R_2/(R_1 + R_2)$. Thus only when T_1 and T_2 are unequal is there a frequency dependency of C_{dyn} and R_{dyn}. Since C_{dyn} can be measured statically (f = 0) whereas R_{dyn} is limited to breathing frequencies, a better assessment of frequency dependence is provided by C_{dyn} measurements. Woolcock and co-workers (*17*) maintain that measurement of frequency dependence of C_{dyn} can be used as an index of peripheral airway obstruction. Thus this test appears to be a sensitive test of airways dysfunction, but the requirement of swallowing an esophageal balloon limits its application.

Mechanical Function Tests

Conventional lung function tests consist of the measurement of the geometric (volumes), kinematic (flows), and dynamic (resistance and compliance) properties of the lungs as outlined in this chapter. Combined measures such as the forced expiratory volume in one second (FEV_1) or maximum expiratory flow ($\dot{V}_{max}$) at a particular lung volume have also been used. Comparisons of these measured values for a given patient with established normal values (*2, 7*) are then made for diagnostic purposes. With the possible exception of the frequency dependence of compliance tests, a limitation of these tests is their relative insensitivity to peripheral airway changes. This is most unfortunate because in chronic obstructive lung disease (emphysema and bronchitis) the site of obstruction to air flow appears to be in the peripheral airways (*7*). Thus early diagnosis of these diseases is difficult if not impossible with conventional tests. One test that is believed to provide an index of peripheral airway resistance is the flow-volume curve. This test consists of plotting air flow vs. volume during a maximum effort expiratory maneuver. Recently, measurements of airway "closing volumes" have also been proposed as a measure of peripheral airway function. This test is simple and rapid and promises to be capable of detecting small airway abnormalities much earlier than the conventional lung function test. We now present the major features of both of these tests.

FLOW VOLUME CURVE

In this test the subject with a noseclip applied is instructed to inspire maximally to TLC (total lung capacity) and follow this with a maximum effort expiration to RV (residual volume). Both flow and volume are measured at the mouth and plotted simultaneously as shown in Figure 3-19. The magnitude of flow at each lung volume is

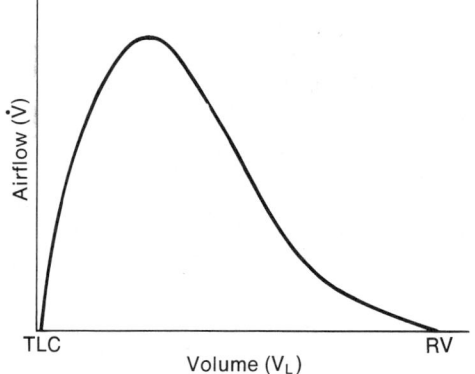

FIGURE 3-19. Maximum expiratory flow-volume curve.

highly effort-dependent at lung volumes near TLC, but as RV is approached, flow is believed to be limited by mechanical properties of the lungs and airways. In order to see how this occurs, let us consider the model shown in Figure 3-20. Shown in the figure is a schematic

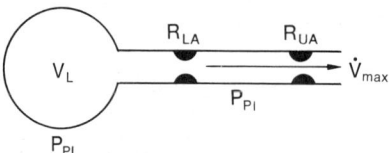

FIGURE 3-20. Schematic representation of the lungs and airways during maximum expiration near TLC.

representation of the lungs (volume V_L) and airways at volumes near TLC, where R_{LA} = lower airway (peripheral) resistance and R_{UA} = upper airway resistance. Pleural pressure (P_{Pl}) surrounds both the lung parenchyma and airways and the alveolar pressure is

$$P_{alv} = P_{Pl} + P_{el} + P_{res}$$

where P_{el} = elastic recoil pressure of the lungs, and
P_{res} = resistive pressure drop due to lung tissue viscosity

For normals, P_{res} is small and can be neglected, leading to the following approximation:

$$P_{alv} \approx P_{Pl} + P_{el}$$

The resultant flow rate with this applied pressure is

$$\dot{V}_{max} = \frac{P_{alv}}{R_{LA} + R_{UA}} \approx \frac{P_{Pl} + P_{el}}{R_{LA} + R_{UA}}$$

Note that the above flow rate is a function of the magnitude of P_{Pl} and is thus effort-dependent. As lung volume approaches RV, P_{Pl} becomes increasingly more positive with respect to intra-airway pressure. A positive P_{Pl} tends to collapse the elastic airways as shown in Figure 3-21. When this collapse occurs, the pressure at the point of collapse

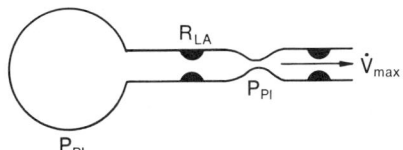

FIGURE 3-21. Schematic representation of the lungs and airways during maximum expiration near RV.

becomes equal to P_{Pl}. The resultant flow rate under this condition is

$$\dot{V}_{max} = \frac{P_{alv} - P_{Pl}}{R_{LA}} \approx \frac{P_{el}}{R_{LA}} \quad (1)$$

Inspection of Figure 3-12 shows that at low lung volumes, the pressure-volume curve of the lungs is quite linear. This justifies the following approximation:

$$P_{el} \approx K_l V_l$$

where K_l = lung elastance.

By substituting the above equation into equation (1), the following approximation results:

$$\dot{V}_{max} \approx \frac{K_1 V_1}{R_{LA}}$$

The above equation shows that the slope of the flow-volume curve near RV is approximately

$$\frac{\Delta \dot{V}}{\Delta V_1} \approx \frac{K_1}{R_{LA}}$$

Thus, the slope of the flow-volume curve near RV is only a function of the elasticity of the lungs and the magnitude of peripheral airway resistance. If peripheral resistance is increased, a flattened flow-volume curve is predicted. This explanation is consistent with the major observations of the flow-volume test in health and disease (1).

CLOSING VOLUME

Dollfuss and associates (6) were the first to study the "closing volume" test of peripheral airway function. Their procedure was as follows: A small bolus (2 to 4 cm^3) of ^{133}xenon was rapidly injected at the mouthpiece during a vital capacity inspiration in human subjects. During the subsequent vital capacity expiration at low constant flow ^{133}xenon concentration was measured at the mouth. In normal subjects the ^{133}xenon concentrations they observed when the bolus was injected near residual volume are shown in Figure 3-22, in which concentration

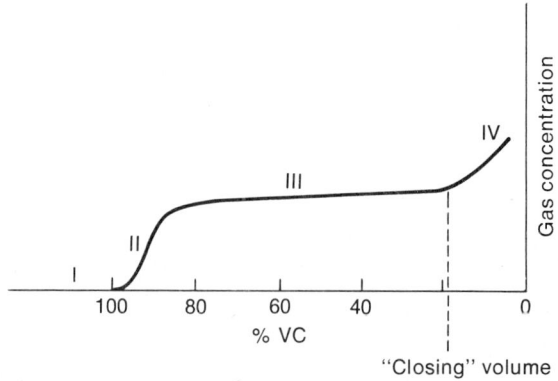

FIGURE 3-22. Expired gas concentration for the *closing volume* maneuver (normal).

is plotted as a function of lung volume. The resultant curve can be separated into four major phases as shown in the figure. After the dead space washout (see Chapter 4) (I and II), a slowly rising curve follows (III), and finally a sharp slope increase is observed at low lung volumes (IV). Similar curves result for bolus injections of helium (3) and argon (9). Also, if a vital capacity inspiration of 100% oxygen is used, the nitrogen washout follows the same shape (8). The lung volume at which the sharp slope increase in concentration is observed is defined as *closing volume*. This "volume" is apparently independent of the gas used in its determination (8). In 66 normal subjects, McCarthy and associates (9) have found "closing volume" to increase with age in the following way:

"closing volume" (% VC) = 1.9 + 0.36 × age (years)

The above regression was based on seated subjects and argon boli. In general, small airway abnormality is associated with an increase in "closing volume" or a grossly different shape in the expired gas-lung volume curve such as shown in Figure 3-23. Such increases in "closing volume" or "curve abnormality" are observed in smokers (5) or patients with chronic obstructive lung disease (8). Let us now consider the possible factors responsible for the above behavior.

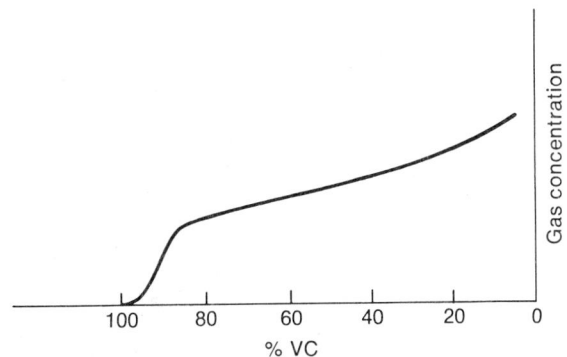

FIGURE 3-23. Expired gas concentration for the *closing volume* maneuver (abnormal).

The simplified model we shall apply is shown in Figure 3-24. The upright human lung is divided into an upper and a lower region each with a separate airway that ultimately merges. If we assume a TLC (total lung capacity) of 8 liters, the upper and lower regions will each consist of 4 liters of regional TLC. There is a gravity-dependent

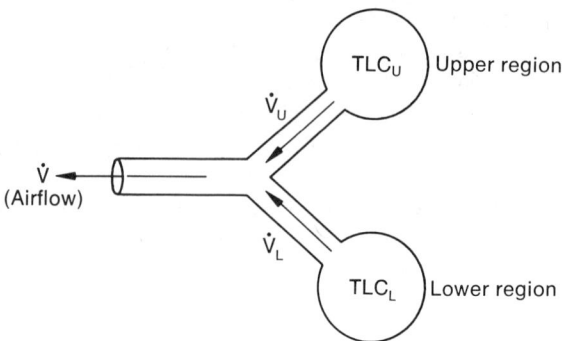

FIGURE 3-24.   Simplified lung model.

gradient in pleural pressure from the lung apex to the base of the order of 0.2 cm H_2O/cm descent in the lungs (*10*). Thus the lower lung region has on the order of 4 to 5 cm H_2O higher pleural pressure than the upper region. The subatmospheric pleural pressure would then be decreased in magnitude at the lower region by 4 to 5 cm H_2O. This means that if lung tissue elasticity is uniform for the upper and lower regions, then the upper region for a given total lung volume will have a larger volume than the lower until TLC is reached. Radioactive gas studies (*10*) show that apical RV is about twice that of basal (RV_U = RV_L). If we assume that (*3*)

$$RV = \frac{TLC}{4} = 2.0 \text{ liters}$$

then the upper and lower region RV's would be

$$RV_L = \tfrac{2}{3} \text{ liter}$$
$$RV_U = \tfrac{4}{3} \text{ liter}$$

Let us now follow the sequence of events in a "closing volume" maneuver using N_2. From RV, a vital capacity inspiration of 100% O_2 results in the following N_2 concentrations:

$$\% \ N_2 \text{ (upper lobe)} = \frac{N_2 \text{ in } RV_U}{TLC_U} \times 100 = \frac{(79)(4/3)}{4} = 26$$

$$\% \ N_2 \text{ (lower lobe)} = \frac{(79)(2/3)}{4} = 13$$

Note that the upper lobe N_2 concentration is double that of the lower

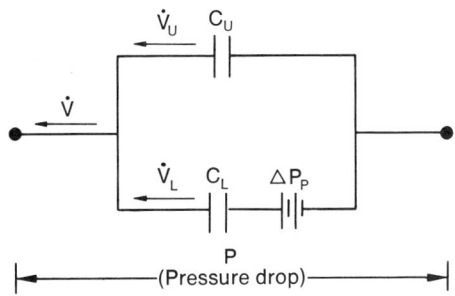

FIGURE 3-25. Electrical analog of lung elasticity.

region. At low expired flow levels, the resistive pressure drops will be small and flows from the two regions are largely determined by regional compliance. This is easily seen from an electrical analog representation of Figure 3-24 as shown in Figure 3-25. The common pressure drop is

$$P = \frac{V_U}{C_U} = \Delta P_{Pl} + \frac{V_L}{C_L}$$

where C_U and C_L are regional compliances and ΔP_{Pl} is the gravity-dependent difference in pleural pressure between upper and lower regions. By differentiating P with respect to time,

$$\dot{P} = \frac{\dot{V}_U}{C_U} = \frac{\dot{V}_L}{C_L}$$

By rewriting the above equation,

$$\frac{\dot{V}_U}{\dot{V}_L} = \frac{C_U}{C_L}$$

For a constant total expired flow ($\dot{V} = \dot{V}_U + \dot{V}_L$),

$$\dot{V}_L = \dot{V}\frac{C_L}{C_U + C_L}$$

$$\dot{V}_U = \dot{V}\frac{C_U}{C_U + C_L}$$

Thus the relative magnitude of regional compliance is the primary determinant of regional flow when all airways are open. If $C_U = C_L$, then $\dot{V}_L = \dot{V}_U = \dot{V}/2$ and the expired N_2 concentration is

$$\frac{26 + 13}{2} = 19.5\%$$

If $C_L = C_U/2$, then $\dot{V}_L$ would provide only a third of the total flow and

$$\% \; N_2 = \tfrac{1}{3}(13) + \tfrac{2}{3}(26) = 21.7$$

The rise of pleural pressure during progressive expiration tends to lead to airway collapse. Since pleural pressure is closer to atmospheric pressure in the lower region, these units should close first. Closure of lower region units would lead to an increase in expired N_2 concentration. In the limit, if the entire lower region were closed, the expired N_2 concentration would rise to 26%. Thus the following explanation can now be given of the expired N_2–lung volume curve during a "closing volume" maneuver: With reference to Figure 3-22, phase III can be caused by changes in relative magnitude of regional compliance with C_L decreasing more rapidly than C_U as RV is approached. Finally, phase IV can occur when lower airway closure occurs progressively, which leads to a rapid increase in N_2 concentration. Abnormal emptying patterns, such as shown in Figure 3-23, can be explained by large changes in regional compliance and/or increase in the volume range over which airway closure occurs. At the present time it is not definitely known whether or not true airway closure occurs. However, the above explanation appears adequate to explain the major observations up to now.

References

1. Bass, H. The flow volume loop: Normal standards and abnormalities in chronic obstructive pulmonary disease. *Chest* **63**: 171–176, 1973.
2. Bates, D. V., P. T. Macklem, and R. V. Christie. *Respiratory Function in Disease*. Philadelphia: W. B. Saunders Co., 1971.
3. Briscoe, W. A. Lung volumes. In: *Handbook of Physiology*, Section 3, *Respiration*, Vol. 2. Edited by W. O. Fenn and H. Rahn. Washington, D.C.: American Physiological Society, 1965, pp. 1345–1379.
4. Brown, E. S., R. P. Johnson, and J. A. Clements. Pulmonary surface tension. *J. Appl. Physiol.* **14**: 717–720, 1959.
5. Buist, S., D. Van Fleet, and B. B. Ross. A comparison of conventional spirometric tests and the test of closing volume in an emphysema screening center. *Am. Rev. Respir. Dis.* **107**: 735–743, 1973.
6. Dollfuss, R. E., J. Milic-Emili, and D. V. Bates. Regional ventilation of the lung studied with boluses of ^{133}xenon. *Respir. Physiol.* **2**: 234–246, 1967.

7. Knudson, R. J., and B. Burrows. Early detection of obstructive lung diseases. *Med. Clin. North Am.* **57:** 681–690, 1973.
8. Linn, W. S., and J. D. Hackney. Nitrogen and helium "closing volumes": Simultaneous measurement and reproducibility. *J. Appl. Physiol.* **34:** 396, 1973.
9. McCarthy, D. S., R. Spencer, R. Greene, and J. Milic-Emili. Measurement of "closing volume" as a simple and sensitive test for early detection of small-airway disease. *Am. J. Med.* **52:** 747–753, 1972.
10. Milic-Emili, J., J. A. M. Henderson, M. B. Dolovich, D. Trop, and K. Kaneko. Regional distribution of inspired gas in the lung. *J. Appl. Physiol.* **21:** 749–759, 1966.
11. Milic-Emili, J., J. Mead, J. M. Turner, and E. M. Glauser. Improved technique for estimating pleural pressure from esophageal balloons. *J. Appl. Physiol.* **19:** 207–211, 1964.
12. Neergaard, K. von. Neue Auffassungen über einen Grundbegriff der Atemmechanik. Die Retraktionskraft der Lunge, abhängig von der Oberflächenspannung in den Alveolen. *Z. Ges. Exp. Med.* **66:** 373–394, 1929.
13. Otis, H. B., C. B. McKerrow, R. A. Bartlett, J. Mead, M. B. McIlroy, N. J. Selverstone, and E. P. Radford, Jr. Mechanical factors in distribution of pulmonary ventilation. *J. Appl. Physiol.* **8:** 427–443, 1956.
14. Radford, E. P., Jr. Recent studies of mechanical properties of mammalian lungs. In: *Tissue Elasticity.* Edited by J. W. Remington. Washington, D. C.: American Physiological Society, 1957, pp. 177–190.
15. Rohrer, F. Physiologie der atembewegung. In: *Handbuch der Normalen und Pathologischen Physiologie*, Vol. 2. Edited by A. Bethe et al. Berlin: Springer-Verlag, 1925, pp. 70–127.
16. Turner, J. M., J. Mead, and M. E. Wohl. Elasticity of human lungs in relation to age. *J. Appl. Physiol.* **25:** 664–671, 1968.
17. Woolcock, A. J., N. J. Vincent, and P. T. Macklem. Frequency dependence of compliance as a test for obstruction in the small airways. *J. Clin. Invest.* **48:** 1097–1106, 1969.

CHAPTER

The Pulmonary Gas Exchanger

Introduction

THE JOB OF THE PULMONARY GAS EXCHANGER is to bring fresh air and stale blood into juxtaposition across a thin (0.5 μm) diffusion membrane so that O_2 and CO_2 transfer can take place between them. Neither all of the "fresh" air inspired nor all of the "stale" systemic venous blood pumped by the heart reaches this effective exchange surface, estimated to total 90 m^2, even in normal people. In disease, this "inefficiency" of ventilation and/or perfusion may be greatly magnified.

Thus the fresh air that is inspired must traverse a treelike arrangement of conducting airways to reach the alveoli where gas exchange with the blood occurs by diffusion. The single trachea leads into some 23 sequential generations of dichotomous branching as summarized in Figure 4-1 and Tables 4-1 and 4-2. Generations 0 through 16 are purely conducting, 17 through 19 are partly conducting and partly diffusing, and 20 through 23 are all diffusing airways. There are two ways in which the inspired air can avoid participating in gas exchange with the blood: (1) it can remain in the conducting airway (i.e., generations 0 to 16) and, obviously, some of it always does, or (2) it can reach nonperfused alveoli. In analogous fashion, there are two ways in which the systemic venous blood can avoid participating in gas exchange with the inspired air: (1) it can pass through anatomic channels that bypass the alveoli completely (e.g., part of the venous return from the bron-

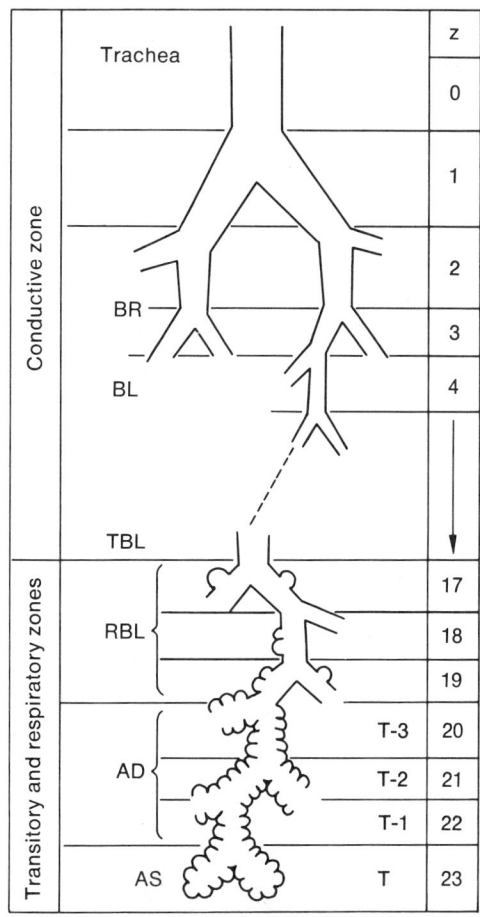

FIGURE 4-1. General architecture of conductive and transitory airways: z designates the order of generation of branching, T the terminal generation. (From E. R. Weibel. *Morphometry of the Human Lung.* Heidelberg: Springer-Verlag; New York: Academic Press, Inc., 1963.)

chial circulation normally goes directly to the left atrium via the pulmonary veins), or (2) it can reach nonventilated alveoli (Figure 4-2).

If we call the total volume of air inspired per minute $\dot{V}_I$, then we can call that portion remaining in the conducting airway $\dot{V}_{cds}$ (conductive dead space ventilation), and the rest, which reaches the alveoli, $\dot{V}_A$ (the alveolar ventilation). That portion of $\dot{V}_A$ that reaches nonperfused alveoli we can call $\dot{V}_{Ads}$ (alveolar dead space ventilation) and the rest, which reaches perfused alveoli and undergoes gas exchange with the blood, $\dot{V}_e$ (effective ventilation). During expiration, expired effective air mixes with alveolar dead air to form expired alveolar air, and this in

TABLE 4-1
Dimensions of Human Airway Model "A"
Average Adult Lung with Volume 4,800 ml at About $\frac{3}{4}$ Maximal Inflation*

Generation z	Number per Generation n(z)	Diameter d(z) (cm)	Length l(z) (cm)	Total Cross Section S(z) (cm²)	Total Volume V(z) (cm³)	Accumulated Volume $\sum_{i=0}^{z} V(i)$ (cm³)
0	1	1.8	12.0	2.54	30.50	30.5
1	2	1.22	4.76	2.33	11.25	41.8
2	4	0.83	1.90	2.13	3.97	45.8
3	8	0.56	0.76	2.00	1.52	47.2
4	16	0.45	1.27	2.48	3.46	50.7
5	32	0.35	1.07	3.11	3.30	54.0
6	64	0.28	0.90	3.96	3.53	57.5
7	128	0.23	0.76	5.10	3.85	61.4
8	256	0.186	0.64	6.95	4.45	65.8
9	512	0.154	0.54	9.56	5.17	71.0
10	1,024	0.130	0.46	13.4	6.21	77.2
11	2,048	0.109	0.39	19.6	7.56	84.8
12	4,096	0.095	0.33	28.8	9.82	94.6
13	8,192	0.082	0.27	44.5	12.45	106.0
14	16,384	0.074	0.23	69.4	16.40	123.4
15	32,768	0.066	0.20	113.0	21.70	145.1
16	65,536	0.060	0.165	180.0	29.70	174.8
17	131,072	0.054	0.141	300.0	41.80	216.6
18	262,144	0.050	0.117	534.0	61.10	277.7
19	524,288	0.047	0.099	944.0	93.20	370.9
20	1,048,576	0.045	0.083	1,600.0	139.50	510.4
21	2,097,152	0.043	0.070	3,220.0	224.30	734.7
22	4,194,304	0.041	0.059	5,880.0	350.00	1,084.7
23*	8,388,608	0.041	0.050†	11,800.0	591.00	1,675.0

*From E. R. Weibel, *Morphometry of the Human Lung*. New York: Academic Press, Inc., and Heidelberg, Germany: Springer-Verlag, 1963.
† Adjusted for complete generation.

turn mixes with conductive dead air to form expired air, $\dot{V}_E$. Note that the only portion of $\dot{V}_I$ that changes its composition between inspiration and expiration is the effective portion, $\dot{V}_e$.

A closely analogous description applies to the blood flow. If we call the total flow rate of systemic venous blood $\dot{Q}_v$, then we can call that portion which bypasses the alveoli completely $\dot{Q}_{cs}$, the conductive shunt flow (e.g., part of the bronchial venous return), and the rest, that which reaches the alveolar capillary network, $\dot{Q}_A$, the alveolar capillary flow. That portion of $\dot{Q}_A$ which reaches nonventilated alveoli we call $\dot{Q}_{As}$ (alveolar shunt flow), and the rest, which reaches ventilated alveoli and undergoes gas exchange with the effective air, we call $\dot{Q}_e$ (effective

TABLE 4-2
Numerical Values of Respiratory Zone Model for Average Adult*

Component	Value
Volume of model lung	4800 ml
Volume of respiratory zone	3150 ml
Volume of capillary network	140 ml
Number of alveoli	$300 \cdot 10^6$
Air-tissue interface	$95 \; m^2$
Tissue-blood interface	$90 \; m^2$
Radius of alveolus	$140 \; \mu m$
Volume of alveolus	$10.5 \cdot 10^{-6} \; cm^3$
Surface of alveolus	$30 \cdot 10^{-4} \; cm^2$
Number of capillary segments per alveolus	1800
Capillary blood volume per alveolus†	$4.7 \cdot 10^{-7} \; cm^3$
Capillary surface per alveolus†	$28 \cdot 10^{-4} \; cm^2$
Radius of capillary segments	$4 \cdot 10^{-4} \; cm$
Mean length of capillary segments	$10.3 \cdot 10^{-4} \; cm$

*From E. R. Weibel, *Morphometry of the Human Lung.* New York: Academic Press, Inc., and Heidelberg, Germany: Springer-Verlag, 1963.

† Refers to the half network belonging to the alveolus (cf. text).

blood flow). After having undergone gas exchange (which changes its O_2 and CO_2 levels from those of "mixed venous" to those of "effective" or "end capillary blood," ec), the effective blood flow mixes with the conductive and alveolar shunt flows in the left heart to form arterial blood. Note again that the only portion of $\dot{Q}_v$ which changes its composition before entering the left heart is the effective portion, $\dot{Q}_e$. Oxygen and CO_2 exchange between effective air and effective blood takes place by a process of passive diffusion, and, normally, complete diffusion equilibrium is achieved for both gases so that after exchange, $P_{eCO_2} = P_{ecCO_2}$ and $P_{eO_2} = P_{ecO_2}$. In normal people at rest, about 25% of $\dot{V}_I$ is wasted as $\dot{V}_{cds}$, whereas only about 2% of $\dot{Q}_v$ is wasted as $\dot{Q}_{cs}$. Also, in normal people, $\dot{V}_{Ads} = 0 = \dot{Q}_{As}$; i.e., there is normally neither a true alveolar dead space nor a true alveolar shunt.

We can conveniently summarize this description of air and blood flow through the pulmonary gas exchanger in the form of a table (Table 4-3) that gives both flow rates and compositions for a normal man at rest. The compositions given for effective air and effective blood are those after gas exchange has occurred. Before this exchange, effective air has the same composition as tracheal air, and effective blood has the same composition as mixed venous blood. In addition to the general summary that Table 4-3 provides, it also illustrates several special

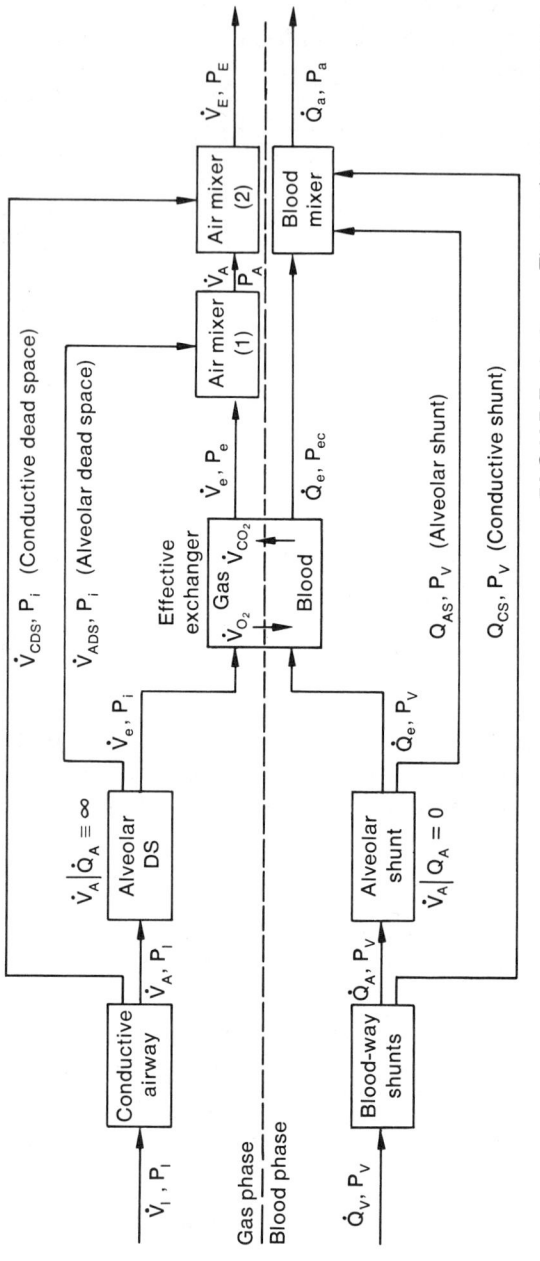

FIGURE 4-2. The exchange apparatus.

TABLE 4-3

Phase	Subscript Symbol	Flow Rate L/min	CO$_2$ P	CO$_2$ C	O$_2$ P	O$_2$ C	N$_2$ P	N$_2$ C	H$_2$O P	H$_2$O C	Total Tension
I. Gas Phase											
a. Inspired air											
(1) Dry	—	6.43	0	0	160	21	600	79	0	0	760
(2) Wet ≡ tracheal air	—	6.85	0	0	150	19.7	563	74	47	6.2	760
b. Conductive DS air	cds	1.80	0	0	150	19.7	563	74	47	6.2	760
c. Alveolar DS air	Ads	0.00	0	0	150	19.7	563	74	47	6.2	760
d. Effective air	e	5.00	40	5.3	103	13.5	570	75	47	6.2	760
e. Expired alveolar air	EA	5.00	40	5.3	103	13.5	570	75	47	6.2	760
f. Expired air (wet)	E	6.80	30	4.0	115	15.1	568	74.7	47	6.2	760
II. Blood Phase											
a. Mixed venous blood	v	6.00	47	52.9	40	15.7	570	1	47	—	704
b. Conductive shunt blood	cs	0.10	47	52.9	40	15.7	570	1	47	—	704
c. Alveolar shunt blood	As	0.00	47	52.9	40	15.7	570	1	47	—	704
d. Effective blood	e*	5.90	40	49	103	20.4	570	1	47	—	760
e. Arterial blood	a	6.00	40	49	95	20.3	570	1	47	—	752

$\dot{V}_{O_2} = 0.275$ L/min $\dot{V}_{CO_2} = 0.234$ L/min   RQ = 0.85

* e (flow) or ec (gas tension).

features; e.g., because R is less than 1, expired volume (6.80) is slightly less than inspired volume (6.85) and expired N_2 content (74.7%) slightly higher than inspired N_2 (74%). Note also that whereas the normal 2% conductive shunt flow does not affect the equality of $P_{e_{CO_2}}$ and $P_{a_{CO_2}}$, it does cause an 8 mm Hg difference for P_{O_2}. This has to do with differences in the shapes of the CO_2 and O_2 dissociation curves, which we shall consider later. Another consequence of this difference is the large drop in venous P_{O_2} and the relatively small rise in P_{CO_2} that accompany tissue gas exchange. This inequality leads to a total gas tension in venous blood that is considerably below ambient barometric pressure and provides a gradient for the absorption of gas from body tissues or cavities.

With this overall introduction, let us now examine the operation of the gas exchanger in more detail. We begin with the gas phase, first examining the conducting airway and the partition of $\dot{V}_I$ into $\dot{V}_{cds}$ and $\dot{V}_A$.

Gas Phase

THE CONDUCTIVE AIRWAY

Let us divide the total lung volume into two parts: (1) the conducting airway and (2) the alveolar space. The former includes generations 0 to 16 of Weibel and the latter generations 20 to 23, with the transition zones 17 to 19 shared between them. Let us begin by assuming that at the resting expiratory position, i.e., at FRC, the geometric volume of the conducting airways is 180 ml and that of the alveolar space is 2320 ml. Now consider the simplest possible division of an inspired tidal volume of 685 ml between these two parts. If the inspired air traveled in plug fashion (i.e., square front) through the airways and if the only volume expansion occurred in the alveolar space, then 180 ml of the inspired V_T would occupy the conducting airway and the rest (505 ml) would reach the alveolar space. Unfortunately, neither of these simplifying assumptions is true. The volume of the conducting airway increases with tidal volume and the inspired air flow is laminar with a parabolic front. The former alone would increase the volume of inspired air remaining in the conducting airway, whereas the latter alone would decrease it because the effective cross section for laminar flow is less than the actual anatomic cross section. How can we best include such features in our description of the partition of $\dot{V}_I$?

Let us note first that we can express this partition in functional rather than anatomical terms by defining the component volumes on the basis of their gas composition rather than as anatomic spaces. Assuming for the moment that we are dealing with a normal person with no alveolar dead space, we can say that the total expired tidal volume, V_T, represents a mixture of two components. One, the conductive dead space volume, V_{cds}, has the composition of inspired air, F_I, and the other, the alveolar or effective volume V_A (or V_e), has the composition of effective air, F_e. Hence for total volume:

$$V_T = V_{cds} + V_A \tag{1}$$

and for any given gas

$$F_E V_T = F_I V_{cds} + F_e V_A \tag{2}$$

where the F's are the appropriate fractions of that gas in expired, inspired, and effective volumes, respectively. Combining (1) and (2) yields the "Bohr formulas" for the virtual (i.e., defined by gas composition rather than morphology) volumes, V_{cds} and V_A:

$$V_{cds} = \frac{F_e - F_E}{F_e - F_I} V_T \tag{3}$$

$$V_A = \frac{F_E - F_I}{F_e - F_I} V_T \tag{4}$$

Since it is easy to measure V_T, F_I, and F_E, we could calculate V_{cds} and V_A if we could measure F_e. In normal people where $F_e = F_A$ (i.e., $V_{Ads} = 0$), we can measure F_e from an alveolar sample. There are two principal methods for obtaining such samples. The older Haldane method takes the last portion of a deep expiration. Although this minimizes the risk of contaminating V_A with V_{cds}, it alters the normal cycle in the direction of hypoventilation so that F_{CO_2} may be too high and F_{O_2} too low, an effect that increases with metabolic rate. The Rahn method samples the last portion of a normal expiration (end tidal sample), thus preserving the normal cycle but risking contamination with V_{cds}. Since the composition of effective air is, in fact, neither uniform in space nor steady in time, both methods aim to achieve some sort of appropriate spatial and temporal average. A better method than either of these, if arterial puncture is not out of the question, is to measure $P_{a_{CO_2}}$ (*vide infra*).

Thus we have operational definitions that allow us to measure the partition of V_T into V_{cds} and V_A (or V_e). It is convenient to express this partition in terms of an "alveolar fraction," AF, which we define as the ratio of V_A ($=V_e$ in normal persons) to V_T:

$$AF = \frac{V_A}{V_T} = \frac{V_e}{V_T} \tag{5}$$

and it is clear from equation (4) that this can be easily calculated as the ratio of F_{ECO_2} to F_{ACO_2} (or P_{ECO_2}/P_{ACO_2}), since $F_{ICO_2} = 0$, and $F_{eCO_2} = F_{ACO_2}$. Using the appropriate figures from Table 4-3, its normal value is 30/40 or 0.75. We can call (1 − AF) the "physiologic conductive dead space fraction," which is thus normally about 0.25.

What are the important factors that determine the value of AF? From our earlier discussion, it is clear that the critical one is the relative size of the "functional conductive dead space" and the tidal volume. It is easy to measure the tidal volume, but what is the relationship between the "functional" (or physiologic) conductive dead space and its anatomic counterpart? We know that the size of the anatomic dead space increases with lung volume, whereas the nature of laminar flow "wash-out" reduces its functional size. It turns out that both of these effects can be described by a model comprising a virtual cylindrical dead space washed out by laminar flow during expiration. Thus we define the virtual dead space, DS, as that virtual cylindrical space which, if filled with inspired air at the beginning of expiration and then washed out by laminar flow, would yield the observed V_{cds} by the Bohr formula [equation (3)]. The virtual dead space so defined is a linear function of tidal volume, V_T:

$$DS = 180 + 0.023\, V_T \tag{6}$$

and the physiologic conductive dead space that it yields is defined by the laminar washout equation:

$$V_{cds} = DS\left(1 - \frac{DS}{4V_T}\right) \tag{7}$$

and the corresponding alveolar fraction by

$$AF = \left(1 - \frac{DS}{2V_T}\right)^2 \tag{8}$$

Equation (8) is plotted in Figure 4-3, which shows that AF = 0 when $V_T = DS/2$ and rises to a limiting asymptotic value of 1 when V_T gets very large. Any increase in DS shifts the entire curve to the right giving lower values for AF at any given V_T.

THE ALVEOLAR DEAD SPACE

So far we have assumed that we were dealing with a normal subject in whom $V_{Ads} = 0$ so that $V_A = V_e$ and $F_A = F_e$. It is "easy" under these conditions to partition V_E into two functional components based on gas composition as we have just done. But suppose now that we are dealing with a patient in whom $V_{Ads} \neq 0$. What this means is that some of the inspired gas that reaches the alveolar space goes to nonperfused

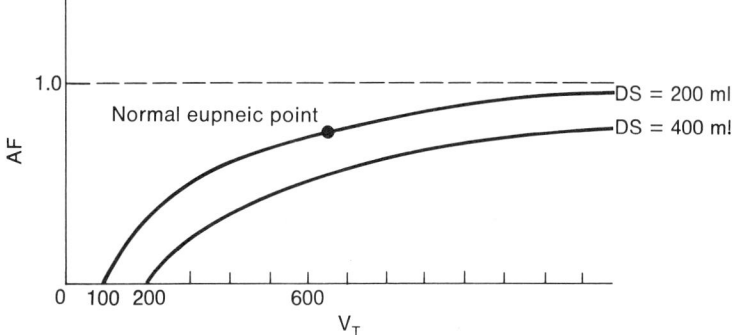

FIGURE 4-3. Alveolar fraction (AF) versus tidal volume (V_T) for two fixed values of virtual dead space (DS).

alveoli and so does not undergo gas exchange with pulmonary capillary blood. Thus, like air that remains in the conductive dead space, this portion of the alveolar gas retains the composition of inspired air and comprises a functional alveolar dead space. Such a situation might occur, for example, if a pulmonary embolus blocked blood flow to part of the lung. How can we functionally partition the total tidal volume under these conditions?

In principle the problem is no different from the one we have just solved. Thus we can first partition the total quantity of a given gas in the expired tidal volume into that contained in V_{cds} and that in V_A just as we did before [cf. equation (2), but now $F_A \neq F_e$]:

$$F_E V_T = F_I V_{cds} + F_A V_A \qquad (9)$$

and then partition the total quantity in V_A into that in V_{Ads} and V_e:

$$F_A V_A = F_I V_{Ads} + F_e V_e \qquad (10)$$

The corresponding total volumes are

$$V_T = V_{cds} + V_A \qquad (11)$$

$$V_A = V_{Ads} + V_e \qquad (12)$$

From these we derive the corresponding "Bohr formulas" for the functional definition of V_{cds}, V_A, V_{Ads}, and V_e:

$$V_{cds} = \left(\frac{F_A - F_E}{F_A - F_I}\right) V_T \qquad (13)$$

$$V_A = \left(\frac{F_E - F_I}{F_A - F_I}\right) V_T \qquad (14)$$

$$V_{Ads} = \left(\frac{F_e - F_A}{F_e - F_I}\right)V_A \tag{15}$$

$$V_e = \left(\frac{F_A - F_I}{F_e - F_I}\right)V_A \tag{16}$$

Again, since it is easy to measure V_E, F_I, and F_E, we could calculate all four component volumes if we could measure F_A and F_e. As we noted before, in a normal subject, $V_{Ads} = 0$, $F_A = F_e$, and an "appropriate" alveolar sample was all that we needed. But now $V_{Ads} \neq 0$, $F_A \neq F_e$, and so we need to measure both. We can get F_A as before from an alveolar sample, but how can we get F_e? Note that unlike V_{cds}, which is a "series" component, V_{Ads} is a "parallel" one. This means that whereas the last portion of V_T is composed of "pure" V_A, all of V_A is a mixture of V_{Ads} and V_e. Hence, it is impossible to determine F_e by sampling any portion of expired gas when $V_{Ads} \neq 0$. What we do instead is to sample arterial blood.

Thus we have already noted that complete diffusion equilibrium is reached in the effective portion of the gas exchanger so that $P_{eCO_2} = P_{ecCO_2}$ and $P_{eO_2} = P_{ecO_2}$. We have also noted that the approximately 2% conductive shunt flow normally present does not significantly alter P_{ecCO_2}, so that $P_{eCO_2} = P_{aCO_2}$, but that this is not true for oxygen. As we shall see later, even an abnormal shunt unless quite large, or a pathologic alveolar membrane diffusion block unless very severe do not produce significant $P_{eCO_2} - P_{aCO_2}$ differences either, nor does a moderate degree of ventilation-perfusion nonuniformity in the effective gas exchanger. Hence we sample arterial blood, determine P_{aCO_2} and define this as P_{eCO_2}.

Once more we have obtained operational definitions and measurable quantities that enable us to partition V_T into V_{cds} and V_A, and to separate V_A into V_{Ads} and V_e. As before, it is convenient to express the first partition in terms of the "alveolar fraction," AF [cf. equation (5)]:

$$AF \equiv \frac{V_A}{V_T} = \frac{F_E - F_I}{F_A - F_I} \tag{17}$$

In an analogous fashion, the second partition can be expressed in terms of an "effective alveolar fraction" (eAF):

$$(eAF) \equiv \frac{V_e}{V_A} = \frac{F_A - F_I}{F_e - F_I} \tag{18}$$

and the overall "effective fraction" (eF) as

$$(eF) \equiv \frac{V_e}{V_T} = (AF)(eAF) = \frac{F_E - F_I}{F_e - F_I} \tag{19}$$

Since we base our calculations on CO_2 and $F_{I_{CO_2}} = 0$, we finally have

$$AF = \frac{F_{E_{CO_2}}}{F_{A_{CO_2}}} = \frac{P_{E_{CO_2}}}{P_{A_{CO_2}}}, \tag{20}$$

$$(eAF) = \frac{F_{A_{CO_2}}}{F_{e_{CO_2}}} = \frac{P_{A_{CO_2}}}{P_{e_{CO_2}}} = \frac{P_{A_{CO_2}}}{P_{a_{CO_2}}} \tag{21}$$

$$(eF) = \frac{F_{E_{CO_2}}}{F_{e_{CO_2}}} = \frac{P_{E_{CO_2}}}{P_{e_{CO_2}}} = \frac{P_{E_{CO_2}}}{P_{a_{CO_2}}} \tag{22}$$

Note that in normal healthy lungs, eAF = 1 and so (eF) = AF. Note also that these fractions apply equally well to a single tidal volume, V_T, or to steady-state ventilation, $\dot{V}$. We used the latter in the summary diagram of Figure 4-2, which you can now refer to again to review our progress so far. Note also that we can call (1 − eAF) the physiologic alveolar dead space fraction and (1 − eF) the total physiologic dead space fraction.

THE EFFECTIVE GAS EXCHANGER

This is the focal point of the whole system, for it is here that the essential function of gas exchange between air and blood takes place. We have already noted that this exchange is accomplished by a process of passive diffusion, and that complete diffusion equilibrium between air and blood is achieved for both O_2 and CO_2, i.e., after exchange $P_{e_{O_2}} = P_{ec_{O_2}}$ and $P_{e_{CO_2}} = P_{ec_{CO_2}}$. Although the exchange process is simple enough in principle, its details are complex and the system can be examined from several different points of view and at various levels of complexity.

If we survey some of these complexities, we note that both the volume and composition of effective gas change continuously with time and space during the respiratory cycle as V_e is inspired and expired. Similarly, the composition of effective blood flowing through the pulmonary capillaries changes with space and time as the blood moves from the entrance to the exit of the capillary. Moreover, both oxygen and carbon dioxide form interrelated chemical combinations with components of blood so that the relation between their blood contents and partial pressures becomes complex and nonlinear. A complete description of these dynamic events in both space and time would require a set of partial differential equations defining air flow, blood flow, and the diffusion process including the nonlinear complexities introduced by the blood chemistry. Such descriptions have been attempted but are beyond the level of our present analysis. Instead, we shall use much simpler models to achieve a useful quantitative understanding of the most essential features of pulmonary gas exchange. Even these simpler models become very awkward to use for practical purposes. Because analytic solutions are difficult or impossible, the early descriptions of the exchange process were often cast in graphic form (10).

By far the simplest way to formulate expressions for the output gas tensions is to deal with the overall, steady-state, mass balance relations for the effective gas phase only. By so doing, we avoid dealing with the details of the diffusion process as well as with the complex, interacting, nonlinear relationships between gas tensions and contents in blood.

What we do is to assume that we know the composition of tracheal air, P_{iO_2} and P_{iCO_2}, the effective ventilation rate, $\dot{V}_e$, and the metabolic oxygen consumption and CO_2 production rates, $\dot{V}_{O_2}$ and $\dot{V}_{CO_2}$. It is then a simple matter to determine what the final gas tensions would be if we added $\dot{V}_{CO_2}$ liters of CO_2 (or subtracted $\dot{V}_{O_2}$ liters of O_2) from $\dot{V}_e$ liters of inspired effective air with initial tensions, P_{iCO_2} and P_{iO_2}:

$$P_{eCO_2} = P_{iCO_2} + \frac{863 \dot{V}_{CO_2}}{\dot{V}_e} \tag{23}$$

and

$$P_{eO_2} = P_{iO_2} - \frac{863 \dot{V}_{O_2}}{\dot{V}_e} \tag{24}$$

The second term on the right in each case represents the change in tension produced by adding $\dot{V}_{CO_2}$ ml (STPD) of CO_2 to (or subtracting $\dot{V}_{O_2}$ ml (STPD) of O_2 from) a constant total volume of $\dot{V}_e$ liters (BTPS). The latter condition (i.e., constancy of $\dot{V}_e$) requires that $\dot{V}_{CO_2} = \dot{V}_{O_2}$, i.e., that $R = RQ = 1$, and when the condition is satisfied, these equations are exactly correct. The equations can be generalized to include any value of R, but they then become extremely awkward in form with only a minimal gain in accuracy. Thus we will assume that equations (23) and (24) are sufficiently accurate for any R over the physiologic range. The constant, 863, reconciles STPD and BTPS units and converts volumetric fraction to partial pressure at sea level (760 × 310/273 = 863).

We can examine the implications of these equations graphically in two revealing ways. First, if we substitute $\dot{V}_{CO_2}/R$ for $\dot{V}_{O_2}$ in (24) it is clear that

$$\frac{863 \dot{V}_{CO_2}}{\dot{V}_e} = (P_{iO_2} - P_{eO_2})R \tag{25}$$

and if we substitute (25) into (23) we have

$$P_{eCO_2} = P_{iCO_2} + RP_{iO_2} - RP_{eO_2} \tag{26}$$

Equation (26) defines a three-parameter family of straight lines relating

P_{eCO_2} to P_{eO_2} for different values of the parameters, R, P_{iO_2}, and P_{iCO_2}. A plot of this family is variously known as the CO_2-O_2 diagram or the alveolar diagram, and representative examples are shown in Figure 4-4. If $P_{iCO_2} = 0$ (which it normally does), the intercept on the P_{eO_2} axis is P_{iO_2}, the slope is R, and the intercept on the P_{eCO_2} axis is RP_{iO_2}. If $P_{iCO_2} > 0$, then each line simply shifts upward P_{iCO_2} mm Hg with no change in slope. Thus the CO_2-O_2 diagram locates all simultaneously compatible values for P_{eCO_2} and P_{eO_2} for any given set of values for P_{iO_2}, P_{iCO_2}, and R. However, it says nothing about which particular pair of values will actually be selected. It turns out that this depends upon the ratio of ventilation to metabolism and this feature is more clearly revealed by a second form of plot.

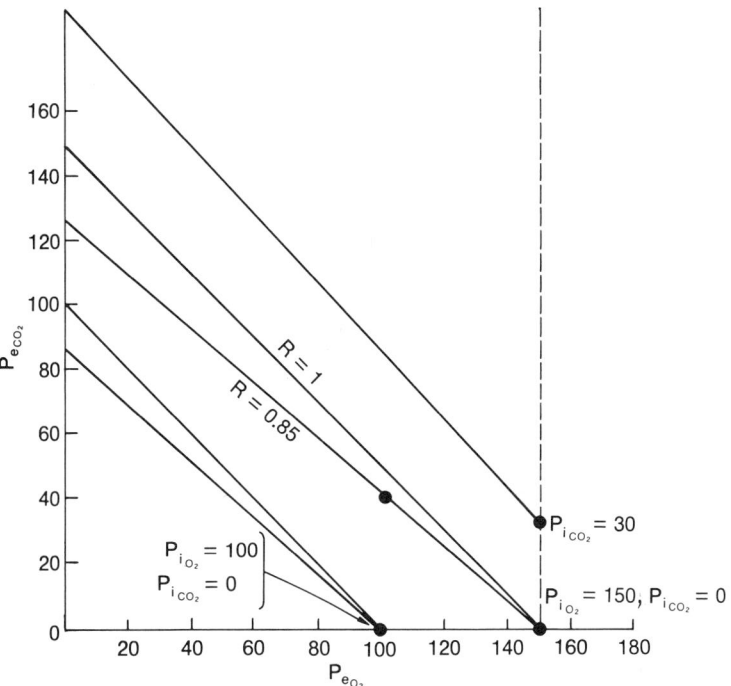

FIGURE 4-4. The CO_2-O_2 alveolar diagram.

Thus, if we define the effective ventilatory equivalent, $\dot{V}_eE$, as the ratio of $\dot{V}_e$ to $\dot{V}_{O_2}$, we can write equations (23) and (24) in the following form:

$$P_{eCO_2} = P_{iCO_2} + \frac{863R}{\dot{V}_eE} \tag{27}$$

$$P_{eO_2} = P_{iO_2} - \frac{863}{\dot{V}_eE} \tag{28}$$

These equations represent families of hyperbolas relating effective gas tensions to $\dot{V}_eE$ for given sets of values of the same parameters as before, P_{iCO_2}, P_{iO_2}, and R. If we take $P_{iCO_2} = 0$, $P_{iO_2} = 150$, and R = 0.85, the corresponding curves are plotted in Figure 4-5. The normal operating points occur at $\dot{V}_eE = 0.183$ where $P_{eO_2} = 103$ and $P_{eCO_2} = 40$. It is now clear that if $\dot{V}_eE$ increases, we move to the right along these curves and P_{eCO_2} falls while P_{eO_2} rises (hyperventilation, hypocapnia, hyperoxia). If $\dot{V}_eE$ falls, we move to the left; P_{eCO_2} rises and P_{eO_2} falls (hypoventilation, hypercapnia, hypoxia). Thus, if we go back to the CO_2-O_2 diagram in Figure 4-3, movement to the left along any curve is brought about by hypoventilation and movement to the right by hyperventilation. Thus these two forms of expression are equivalent but emphasize different features of the basic relations contained in equations (23) and (24).

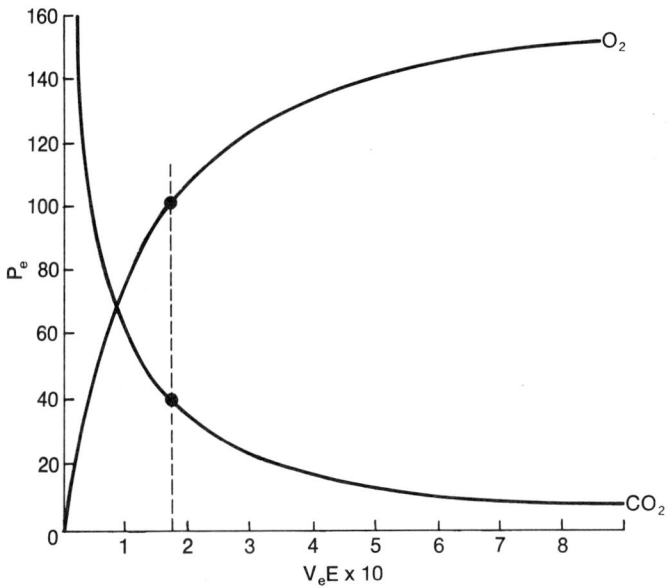

FIGURE 4-5. Effective gas tensions, P_e, versus effective ventilatory equivalent, V_eE. Dashed line intersects normal values for V_eE, P_{eCO_2}, and P_{eO_2}.

We shall consider some of these equations again in still another way when we examine the concept of gas-blood matching. Before we can do this, however, we must first describe the blood phase of the pulmonary gas exchanger.

Blood Phase

We shall be concerned here with the diffusion process across the alveolocapillary membrane as well as with the mixing of effective and shunted blood. To analyze these processes, however, we must understand the physicochemical nature of blood gas transport, and so we begin with this.

BLOOD GASES

In our preview of the gas exchanger we presented normal values for gas tensions in both gas and blood phases. The tension unit is not only common to both phases, it represents the "gradient" that forces diffusion between the two. In the gas phase, tensions are also directly proportional to absolute concentrations (temperature constant), but in the blood phase the relationships between tensions and concentrations are not so simple, and must be examined in detail.

Normal resting values for whole blood gases are presented in Table 4-4. Only *whole blood* concentrations are shown, because they are the significant ones for the gas exchanger (cell and plasma concentrations differ). *Mixed* arterial blood may be sampled from any systemic artery, for the mixing from various pulmonary veins is completed in the left heart; *mixed venous* blood can be sampled (by inserting a catheter) only from the region of the right heart, where mixing from various systemic veins is completed. No values are shown for effective or alveolar blood, since they are not accessible to sampling.

Although blood gas contents (content = concentration) may be expressed in interchangeable units of vol %, or mM/L, we shall use vol % (mM/L × 2.24 = vol %). Blood contains small amounts of *free* gas in simple physical solution, symbolized as (H_2CO_3) and (FO_2). It contains large amounts of *bound* gases, symbolized as (BCO_2), which includes bicarbonate and carbamate forms, and (HbO), as oxyhemoglobin. The sum of the free and bound forms gives the *total* gas contents, symbolized as (CO_2) and (O_2). Although all the O_2 absorbed into the blood in the lungs enters the blood as free O_2, nearly all ends up as bound O_2; the same is true for CO_2 entering the blood in the tissues. Thus the free gas is the *transfer* form and the bound gas the *storage* form. This storage process enormously increases the gas transport capacity of blood.

The *O_2 capacity* of blood is defined as the maximum content of bound O_2, when the blood is exposed (*in vitro*) to a saturating tension of O_2 (air at sea level is adequate). If no inactive Hb is present, each

TABLE 4-4
Normal, Resting Whole Blood Gases*
$(Hbt)b = 15.7 \text{ g\%} \times 1.34 \text{ vol \%/g} = 21.0 \text{ vol \% } O_2 \text{ capacity}$

Whole Blood	Flow L/min	Carbon Dioxide					Oxygen					
		Free		Bound	Total		Free		Bound			Total
		PCO_2	(H_2CO_3)	(BCO_2)	(CO_2)		PO_2	(FO_2)	(HbO)	Sat.		(O_2)
Mixed venous	6	47	2.9	50.0	52.9		43	0.14	15.6	74		15.7
Mixed arterial	6	40	2.5	46.5	49.0		95	0.3	20.0	96		20.3
A-V difference	—	7	0.4	3.5	3.9		52	0.16	4.4	22		4.6

*Tensions in mm Hg, contents in vol %, and saturation in %.

gram of Hb can combine with 1.34 ml of O_2, so that a normal (Hbt) of 15.7 g % yields an O_2 capacity of 21.0 vol %. The O_2 saturation, S, is defined as the ratio of bound O_2 content to O_2 capacity, usually multiplied by 100 to yield a percentage figure. This is a *relative* measure so that for a given % saturation, the bound O_2 may be high or low depending on the O_2 capacity.

For each gas (individually, because of different absorption coefficients), its tension is directly proportional to its free gas content in blood, in accordance with Henry's law. Thus gas tensions become alternate expressions for free gas contents, but *not* for bound or total gas contents. The latter are determined by complex chemical reactions, which we shall examine in a moment.

Return again to Table 4-4 and note that arterial blood retains most of its total CO_2, and venous blood most of its total O_2; the "trucks" are thus only partially unloaded and reloaded with gases as they circulate between the pulmonary and tissue exchangers. Note also the arteriovenous, or A-V, differences included in the table. The A-V difference for P_{CO_2} is only 7 mm Hg, whereas that for P_{O_2} is 52; yet nearly equal amounts of the two gases are exchanged, as shown by their A-V differences for total gas contents. Exchange rates cannot be calculated directly from tensions, but they can easily be calculated from total gas contents as follows:

$$\dot{V}_{O_2} = \frac{\dot{Q}}{100}[(O_2)_a - (O_2)_V] \qquad (29)$$

$$\dot{V}_{CO_2} = \frac{\dot{Q}}{100}[(CO_2)_V - (CO_2)_a] \qquad (30)$$

Total blood gas contents are measured (the blood must be handled anaerobically, i.e., without exposure to air, with which it would otherwise exchange O_2 and CO_2) with a Van Slyke manometric apparatus, which employs a vacuum chamber to extract the total gas from the sample, using acid to liberate bound CO_2 and ferrocyanide to liberate bound O_2; the extracted CO_2 is then measured by absorption with alkali and the O_2 by absorption by pyrogallol; modern methods analyze extracted gases by gas chromatography. Blood gas tensions may be measured by special electrodes applied directly to the blood. From such tensions the free gas contents may be calculated by Henry's law, and bound gases by subtraction from the total.

Now let us turn to the important relationships between gas tensions and total or bound gas contents, known as the *CO_2 dissociation curve* and the *O_2 dissociation curve* (Figure 4-6). Both are chemical equilibrium curves obtained *in vitro* by equilibrating blood aliquots with a

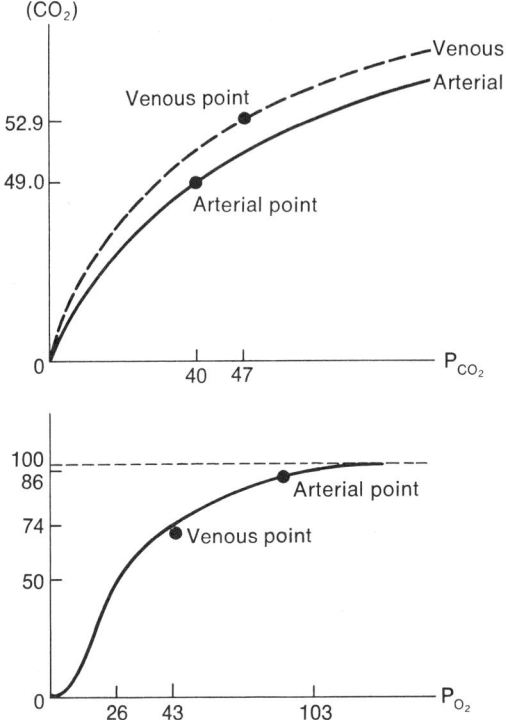

FIGURE 4-6. Above: CO_2 dissociation (or absorption) curve, whole blood CO_2 content, (CO_2), vol. % versus CO_2 tension, P_{CO_2}, mmHg. Below: O_2 dissociation curve, blood O_2 saturation (%) versus O_2 tension, P_{O_2}, mmHg.

series of CO_2, or O_2, tensions, and then measuring the resulting CO_2, or O_2, contents. There is some interaction between the two curves, for the CO_2 curve is appreciably elevated by deoxygenating the blood (the Haldane effect) and the O_2 curve is slightly elevated by decarbonating the blood (the Bohr effect). Also, the addition of alkali will elevate and the addition of acid will lower the CO_2 curve; in discussing the gas exchanger, fortunately, we can ignore this factor. Finally, a high O_2 capacity elevates and a low O_2 capacity lowers the O_2 curve; but if these curves are expressed in terms of O_2 saturation (instead of O_2 content), they merge into one *relative* curve.

The CO_2 absorption curve starts at the origin and rises parabolically (no asymptote) with concavity downward. The normal arterial point ($P_{CO_2} = 40$, $CO_2 = 49$) falls on the oxygenated curve for arterial blood, whereas the normal venous point ($P_{CO_2} = 47$, $CO_2 = 52.9$) falls on the higher, partially deoxygenated curve for venous blood. Since the A-V difference for P_{CO_2} is only 7 mm Hg, the operating range for loading and unloading CO_2 is very narrow.

The O_2 dissociation curve starts at the origin and rises in an asymetrical S-shape to an asymptotic limit of 100% saturation. Half-saturation (P_{50}) occurs at about 22 mm P_{O_2} and full saturation at or above 150 mm Hg. The normal arterial point (P_{O_2} = 95, S = 96%) falls on the partially decarbonated curve for arterial blood, as drawn. The normal venous point (P_{O_2} = 43, S = 74%) is plotted just below the arterial curve; the curve for carbonated venous blood runs too close to plot conveniently. Since the A-V difference for P_{O_2} is 52 mm Hg, the operating range for loading and unloading O_2 is quite wide.

The unique curvature of the O_2 dissociation curve means that the arterial P_{O_2} can fall quite far before the O_2 content or saturation falls appreciably. For example, a P_{O_2} as low as 52 still yields 85% saturation, and one of 45 yields 80% saturation. Unconsciousness supervenes in a few minutes of acute exposure to 60 to 65% arterial saturation, and at this point the P_{O_2} is down to 31 to 34 mm Hg. This is why exposures to altitudes of 10,000 to 15,000 ft are ordinarily so well tolerated—the arterial O_2 content is still adequate for gas transport even though the tension is low.

DIFFUSION PROCESS

Pulmonary diffusion is governed by Fick's law of diffusion:

$$\dot{F}(t) = D \cdot \Delta P(t) \quad \text{in which} \quad D = \frac{Ka}{d} \tag{31}$$

where $\dot{F}(t)$ is the diffusion flux of gas across the membrane at any instant and $\Delta P(t)$ is the gas tension gradient across the membrane at that instant, and this, of course, forces the flux. The coefficient of *diffusance* (commonly called the diffusion capacity), D, depends upon the *diffusivity*, K, of the gas in question, and the area, a, and thickness, d, of the membrane. The relevant gradient across a gas-liquid interface is the tension (not concentration) gradient. Because of its larger molecule, CO_2 diffuses through an aqueous medium only about 75% as fast as O_2 for the same *concentration* gradient; however, because of its 25 times greater solubility, CO_2 diffuses 20 times faster than O_2 for the same *tension* gradient. On this basis alone it has generally been assumed that alveolar pulmonary capillary CO_2 equilibrium is reached very rapidly, much faster than O_2, and that CO_2 elimination, in contrast to O_2 uptake, is not likely to be affected by diffusion difficulties. Recently, however, increasing attention has been given to the role of chemical reaction rates and blood gas capacitances [i.e., Δ(total gas content)/$\Delta P(g)$] in the attainment of gas-blood equilibrium in the lung, and it appears that the older view may need modification.

The following description of the changes in blood gas tensions as the blood traverses the pulmonary capillary networks is based on the predictions of a recent mathematical model that includes chemical reaction rates for O_2 and CO_2 with blood as well as pulmonary diffusing capacity and blood O_2 and CO_2 capacitances in its set of defining equations.

Figure 4-7 plots the time course of P_{O_2} in a particular blood element as it moves down the pulmonary capillary. Although the abscissa is plotted in time units, it could equally well be plotted in length units, and we see that the passage time through the capillary is about 0.75 sec. Mixed venous blood enters the capillary with a P_{O_2} of 40 mm Hg and is immediately exposed to effective air with a P_{O_2} of 100 (assumed constant). Blood P_{O_2} rises rapidly, the plasma slightly leading the red cells until diffusion equilibrium is reached by 0.25 sec, or one third of the capillary transit time. This implies that there is a considerable factor of safety for oxygen diffusion and that capillary transit time can be shortened by 67% before we would expect any dysequilibrium.

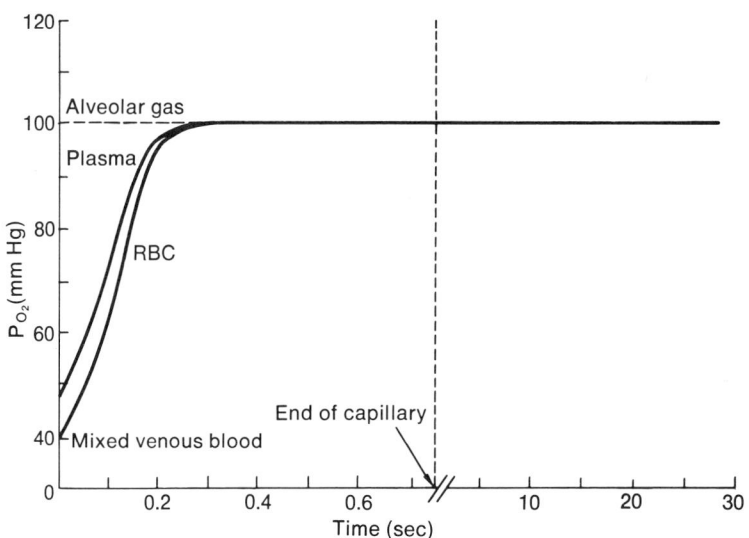

FIGURE 4-7. Normal time course of O_2 partial pressure changes in red cells and plasma during the blood's transit through pulmonary capillaries. Although not important in this particular figure, the right-hand side of each of Figures 4-7 and 4-8 shows changes that occur in arterialized blood after the end of capillary transit. (From E. P. Hill, G. G. Power, and L. D. Longo. Kinetics of O_2 exchange. In: *Bioengineering Aspects of the Lung*. Edited by J. B. West. New York: Marcel Dekker, Inc., 1977.)

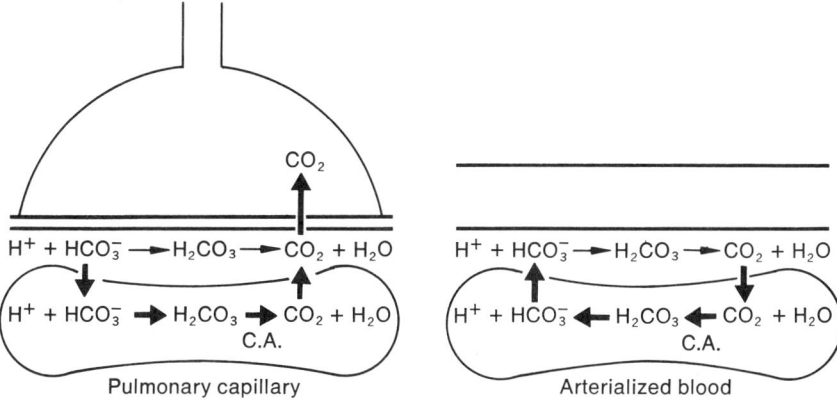

FIGURE 4-10. Diagram showing the main reactions involved in CO_2 elimination during pulmonary capillary transit and reactions that continue after arterialized blood leaves the pulmonary exchange area as plasma approaches chemical equilibrium (see text). (From E. P. Hill, G. G. Power, and L. D. Longo. Kinetics of O_2 exchange. In: *Bioengineering Aspects of the Lung.* Edited by J. B. West. New York: Marcel Dekker, Inc., 1977.)

In pathological diffusion blocks, the graphs would show that the blood gas tensions changed more slowly and might fail to reach the levels in effective air before the blood left the pulmonary capillary.

It is possible to measure the *diffusion capacity,* D_{O_2}, by a difficult and elaborate direct method, or by a simple indirect method that uses carbon monoxide. The subject breathes a low concentration of CO, while its rate of absorption, $\dot{F}_{CO}$, and its alveolar air concentration, $P_{A_{CO}}$ are measured. Under these steady-state conditions, Fick's law reduces to

$$D_{CO} = \frac{\dot{F}_{CO}}{P_{A_{CO}}} \quad \text{then} \quad D_{O_2} = 1.23 D_{CO} \qquad (32)$$

Since the absorbed CO attaches to Hb with enormous affinity, the blood P_{CO}, as it traverses the alveolar capillary, remains essentially zero; hence, the diffusion gradient for the entire traverse is equal to the alveolar P_{CO}. The D_{CO} thus measured is then multiplied by 1.23 to yield the D_{O_2} (the aqueous diffusivity of O_2 is 1.23 times that for CO—the lung geometry is the same for both).

The normal, resting D_{O_2} is about 30 ml/min · mm Hg, but increases in exercise, as previously implied, to 60 or more. It may fall markedly in diffusion block. The rare *berylliosis,* in which the alveolocapillary membrane undergoes fibrotic thickening, is an example of nearly pure diffusion block. Many diseases, however, may reduce the membrane area, or thicken it, including chronic obstructive pulmonary emphysema, and thereby reduce D_{O_2}. Unfortunately, the presence of nonuniform alveoli precludes a meaningful measurement of D_{O_2}, because of difficulty in measuring the precise P_{CO}.

$P_e - P_a$ GRADIENTS. There are three general ways in which $P_e - P_a$ differences can arise. The first, as just described above, is diffusion block brought about by such diseases as berylliosis (rare) or COLD (common), which thicken or reduce the area of the alveolocapillary membrane. The second cause of $P_e - P_a$ gradients is a *blood way shunt*. Normally, about 2% of the cardiac output bypasses the pulmonary gas exchanger through pulmonary A-V shunts, the bronchial venous return, and the Thebesian veins. Because of the nature of the respective dissociation curves, this normal "venous admixture" does not significantly raise P_{aCO_2} but it does lower P_{aO_2} as the following calculations will show:

1. We assume:

$$P_{ecCO_2} = 103 \quad \begin{cases} S_{ec} = 97.1 \\ C_{ecO_2} = 20.4 \end{cases} \quad P_{VO_2} = 43 \quad C_{VO_2} = 15.7$$

$$P_{ecCO_2} = 40 \quad C_{ecCO_2} = 49 \quad P_{VCO_2} = 47 \quad C_{VCO_2} = 52.9$$

2. Then for CO_2:

$$C_{aCO_2} = 0.02(52.9) + 0.98(40) = 49.1 \quad P_{aCO_2} = 40.02$$

and for O_2:

$$C_{aO_2} = 0.02(15.7) + 0.98(20.4) = 20.3; \quad S = 96.6, \quad P_{aO_2} = 95$$

Thus, although P_{aCO_2} is increased by only 0.02 mm Hg, P_{aO_2} is lowered by 8 mm Hg from its end capillary (or effective gas) tension by the normal 2% venous admixture. Similar calculations show that even a 50% shunt (which might occur in congenital heart disease) will only raise P_{aCO_2} by about 3 mm Hg while lowering P_{aO_2} about 43 mm Hg.

The third cause of $P_e - P_a$ gradients is a nonuniformity of gas-blood matching or ventilation-perfusion ratios in the gas exchanger. Our analysis so far has not really admitted this possibility, i.e., our model of the effective gas exchanger has been a lumped homogeneous one with a single gas phase, a single blood phase, and a single $\dot{V}_e/\dot{Q}_e$ ratio. However, since there are some 300 million individual alveoli in the lung, it is highly unlikely that each one would have exactly the same $\dot{V}_e/\dot{Q}_e$ ratio even under normal conditions, let alone in disease. In the latter, the distribution of $\dot{V}_e/\dot{Q}_e$ ratios may include the two extremes of 0 (alveolar shunt) and ∞ (alveolar dead space). We shall analyze the effects of $\dot{V}_e/\dot{Q}_e$ nonuniformity in the next section.

Gas–Blood Matching—The $\dot{V}e/\dot{Q}e$ Ratio

In a previous section we examined some aspects of gas diffusion in the lungs using Fick's equation and noting the changes in gas tensions that occurred as blood moved through the pulmonary capillary. However, although we noted that tension equilibrium was reached between effective air and capillary blood before the latter left the lung, we did not really explain what determined the actual values of these equilibrium tensions. We did previously specify what the equilibrium tensions would be in the effective gas phase of our lumped homogeneous exchanger (see pp. 58–60), but to do this, we used the trick of assuming that we knew what $\dot{V}_{CO_2}$ and $\dot{V}_{O_2}$ were, i.e., that they were independent variables. This is all right for a homogeneous or "ideal" exchanger in the steady state, for then we can measure the relevant $\dot{V}_{CO_2}$ and $\dot{V}_{O_2}$ by expired air analysis and also know that these are the same as metabolic $\dot{V}_{CO_2}$ and $\dot{V}_{O_2}$ and thus that R = RQ. However, this trick effectively excludes any mechanistic role for blood-gas matching and equilibrium constraints in the diffusion process in the lung; i.e., it really does not matter how or from where $\dot{V}_{CO_2}$ was added and $\dot{V}_{O_2}$ subtracted from $\dot{V}_e$. But as soon as we admit the possibility of a nonhomogeneous exchanger, this trick can no longer be used to specify the final gas tensions of mixed effective air and mixed end capillary blood. Instead we must treat the partial $\dot{V}_{CO_2}$ and $\dot{V}_{O_2}$ in each alveolus as the dependent variables that they really are. This greatly complicates our problem, as we shall now see.

Let us look at the beginning and end of the exchange process in a single alveolus. To do this, we expose a certain "minute volume" of wet inspired gas, $\dot{V}_i$, with initial composition $P_{i_{O_2}}$ and $P_{i_{CO_2}}$ to a certain "minute volume" of pulmonary capillary blood, $\dot{Q}_c$, with initial composition $C_{V_{O_2}}$ and $C_{V_{CO_2}}$, and let the two phases exchange O_2 and CO_2 until they reach equilibrium. Clearly, the independent variables here are $\dot{V}_i$, $\dot{Q}_c$, $P_{i_{O_2}}$, $P_{i_{CO_2}}$, $C_{V_{O_2}}$, $C_{V_{CO_2}}$ and the properties of blood, whereas the dependent variables are the exchange rates, $\dot{V}_{O_2}$ and $\dot{V}_{CO_2}$ (and thus the gas exchange ratio, R) and the final concentrations in gas and blood, i.e., $P_{e_{O_2}} = P_{ec_{O_2}}$, $P_{e_{CO_2}} = P_{ec_{CO_2}}$, $C_{ec_{O_2}}$, $C_{ec_{CO_2}}$. The basic principles involved in solving this exchange problem are very simple, involving only mass balance and equilibrium constraints. However, because of the nonlinear and mutually interactive blood dissociation curves for O_2 and CO_2, the solution becomes complex in practice; it was originally cast in a graphic form, which tended to blur the distinction between independent and dependent variables.

We begin the solution by defining all possible equilibrium $P_{O_2} - P_{CO_2}$ combinations for gas and blood by using our already familiar mass balance relations. Thus, for the gas phase, equation (26) defines all possible equilibrium combinations of P_{eCO_2} and P_{eO_2} for given values of R, P_{iO_2}, and P_{iCO_2}. Some examples were plotted in Figure 4-4, but for present purposes we shall use the graph plotted in Figure 4-11. To get corresponding curves for blood, we begin with the

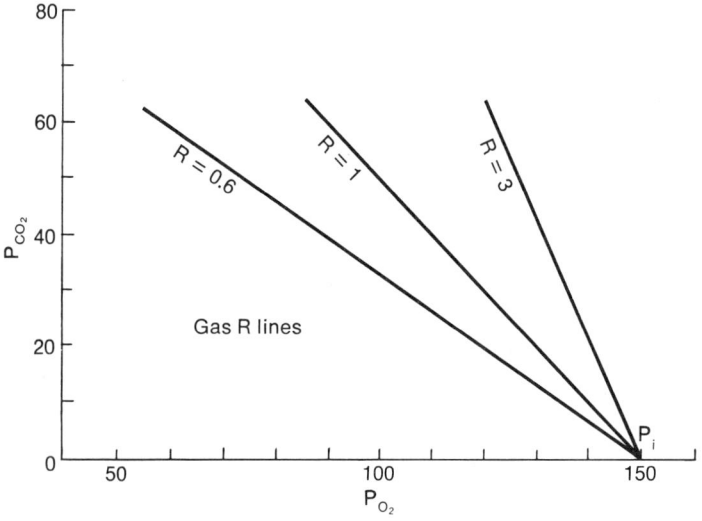

FIGURE 4-11. Gas R lines plotted from equation (26). Isopleths radiating from the inspired air point define all possible values of P_{eO_2} and P_{eCO_2} at the stated value of R.

mass balance equations (29) and (30), which we repeat, slightly modified:

$$\dot{V}_{O_2} = \frac{\dot{Q}_e}{100}(C_{eO_2} - C_{vO_2}) \qquad (33)$$

$$\dot{V}_{CO_2} = \frac{\dot{Q}_e}{100}(C_{vCO_2} - C_{eCO_2}) \qquad (34)$$

Dividing (34) by (33) yields

$$\frac{\dot{V}_{CO_2}}{\dot{V}_{O_2}} \equiv R = \frac{(C_{vCO_2} - C_{eCO_2})}{(C_{eO_2} - C_{vO_2})} \qquad (35)$$

and rearranging,

$$C_{eCO_2} = (C_{VCO_2} + RC_{VO_2}) - RC_{eO_2} \tag{36}$$

Equation (36) defines all possible $C_{eCO_2} - C_{eO_2}$ equilibrium combinations for given values of R and initial blood composition; some examples are plotted in Figure 4-12. Unfortunately, the simple linear relationships in terms of blood gas contents described by equation (36) and plotted in Figure 4-12 cannot be used directly in our

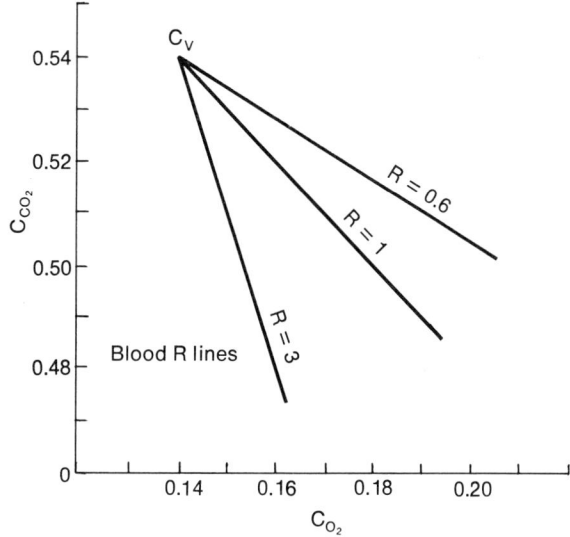

FIGURE 4-12. Blood R lines plotted from equation (36). Isopleths radiating from the mixed venous blood point define all possible values of C_{eO_2} and C_{eCO_2} at the stated value of R.

solution but must first be converted to corresponding curves expressed in terms of blood gas tensions. This translation is done through the nonlinear O_2 and CO_2 dissociation curves, and it is this step that makes the solution complex and nonanalytic. The results of this transformation appear in Figure 4-13.

We can now obtain a simultaneous graphic solution of gas and blood equations by plotting Figures 4-11 and 4-13 on the same graph; this has been done in Figure 4-14. The points of intersection of gas and blood lines for each value of R define the final equilibrium tensions for O_2 and CO_2. We have extrapolated a continuous solution line that defines the equilibrium tensions for other values of R.

74 RESPIRATORY FUNCTION OF THE LUNG AND ITS CONTROL

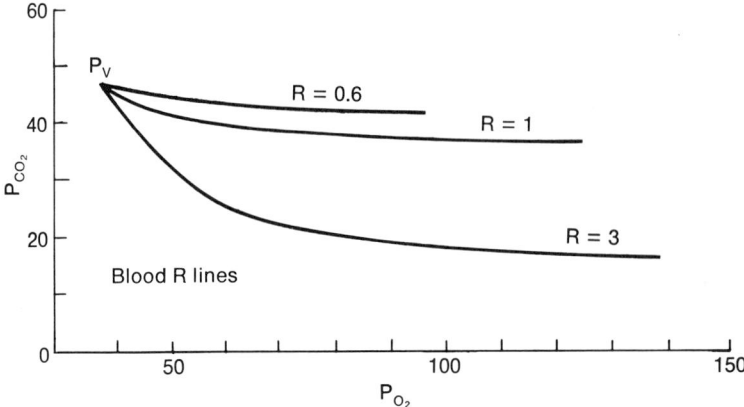

FIGURE 4-13. Blood R lines plotted in terms of partial pressure. The conversion from blood-gas content to partial pressure is made by taking successive points along the blood R lines of Figure 4-12, reading off the corresponding P_{O_2} and P_{CO_2} values from O_2 and CO_2 dissociation curves, and replotting.

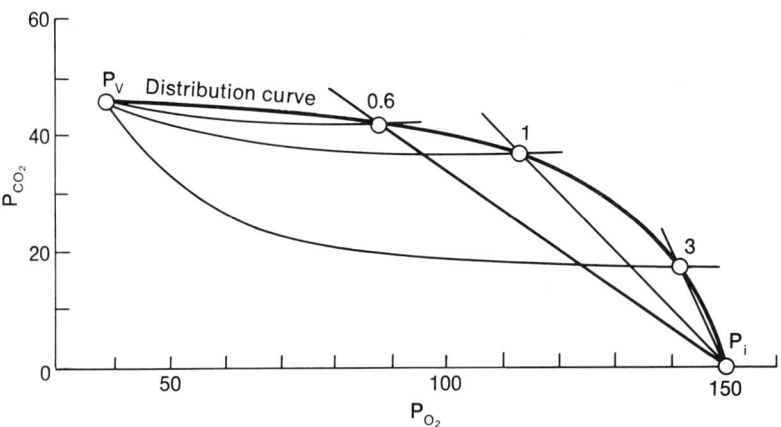

FIGURE 4-14. Blood and gas R lines plotted on the same graph in terms of partial pressure. Points of intersection of blood and gas R lines of equal value are connected to form the "distribution curve."

A somewhat confusing aspect of this form of solution is the fact that R seems to be an independent variable whereas in the actual exchange problem, as we have defined it, R is dependent. However, we can translate each value of R into a corresponding value for the ventilation-perfusion ratio by combining our gas and blood mass balance equations in another way. By dealing with CO_2 exchange only and assuming $P_{i_{CO_2}} = 0$, the gas equation [rearranging equation (23)] is

$$\dot{V}_{CO_2} = \frac{\dot{V}_e P_{e_{CO_2}}}{863} \tag{37}$$

and the blood equation for $\dot{V}_{CO_2}$ [equation (34)] can be written in terms of oxygen concentration differences and R as follows:

$$\dot{V}_{CO_2} = \frac{\dot{Q}_e}{100}(C_{e_{O_2}} - C_{v_{O_2}})R \tag{38}$$

If we now eliminate $\dot{V}_{CO_2}$ between (37) and (38) and solve for $\dot{V}_e/\dot{Q}_e$, we have finally:

$$\frac{\dot{V}_e}{\dot{Q}_e} = \frac{8.63R(C_{e_{O_2}} - C_{v_{O_2}})}{P_{e_{CO_2}}} \tag{39}$$

It should now be clear that for every solution point in Figure 4-14, we know R, $P_{e_{CO_2}}$, $C_{e_{O_2}}$, and $C_{v_{O_2}}$ so that a corresponding value of $\dot{V}_e/\dot{Q}_e$ can be calculated. The results are shown in Figure 4-15, where every point on the solution line now corresponds to a particular $\dot{V}_e/\dot{Q}_e$ ratio, which is in fact one of our independent variables. If the normal $\dot{V}_e/\dot{Q}_e$

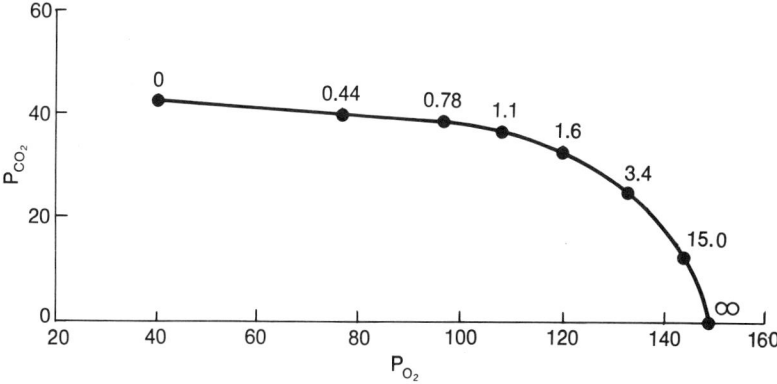

FIGURE 4-15. Ventilation-perfusion ratio or $\dot{V}_A/\dot{Q}$ curve. This line represents all possible gas combinations that can prevail as a result of the equilibration of mixed venous blood with inspired gas. The ratios of ventilation to perfusion responsible for various gas tensions are indicated. These ratios range from 0 representing the mixed venous blood gas tensions to ∞ representing the inspired gas tensions. (From H. Rahn and L. E. Farhi, Ventilation, perfusion, and gas exchange—The $\dot{V}_A/\dot{Q}$ concept. In: *Handbook of Physiology*, Section 3: *Respiration*, Vol. 1. Edited by W. O. Fenn and H. Rahn. Washington, D.C.: American Physiological Society, 1964.)

ratio is 0.85, then movement to the left along the solution line from the normal point represents a decreasing $\dot{V}_e/\dot{Q}_e$ ratio (i.e., hypoventilation) that reaches zero for a true alveolar shunt. Movement to the right from the normal point represents an increasing $\dot{V}_e/\dot{Q}_e$ that reaches infinity for a true alveolar dead space.

One interesting and important result of this analysis is the fact that the final equilibrium gas tensions and the gas exchange ratio depend only upon the ratio of $\dot{V}_e$ to $\dot{Q}_e$ and not upon the absolute value of either. What this says is that if two alveoli have different $\dot{V}_e/\dot{Q}_e$ ratios, their equilibrium gas tensions will differ. Moreover, if after equilibrium has been reached in each alveolus, we separate and then mix the two gas phases and the two blood phases, the resulting mixed gas phase tensions will necessarily differ from the mixed blood tensions. This is because the mixed gas tensions represent a ventilation weighted average whereas the mixed blood tensions represent a perfusion weighted average and the $\dot{V}_e/\dot{Q}_e$ ratios are different for the two alveoli. Thus if gas-blood matching, as measured by the $\dot{V}_e/\dot{Q}_e$ ratio, is not uniform throughout the lung, $P_e - P_a$ gradients can arise from this cause alone. Note that this would be true even though the two extremes of the distribution are not represented, i.e., there need be neither a true alveolar dead space nor a true alveolar shunt.

NONUNIFORMITY IN NORMAL MAN

Recent studies in man using radioactive xenon have shown that both ventilation (Figure 4-16) and blood flow (Figure 4-17) are highest

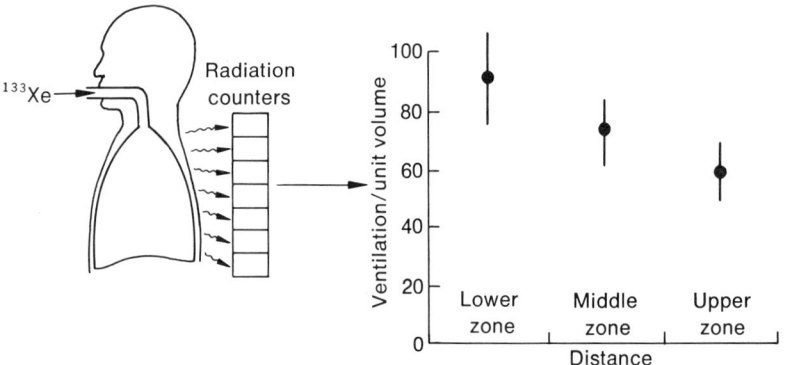

FIGURE 4-16. Measurement of regional differences in ventilation with radioactive xenon. When the gas is inhaled, its radiation can be detected by counters outside the chest. Note that the ventilation decreases from the lower to upper regions of the upright lung. (From J. B. West. *Respiratory Physiology.* Baltimore: The Williams & Wilkins Company, © 1974.)

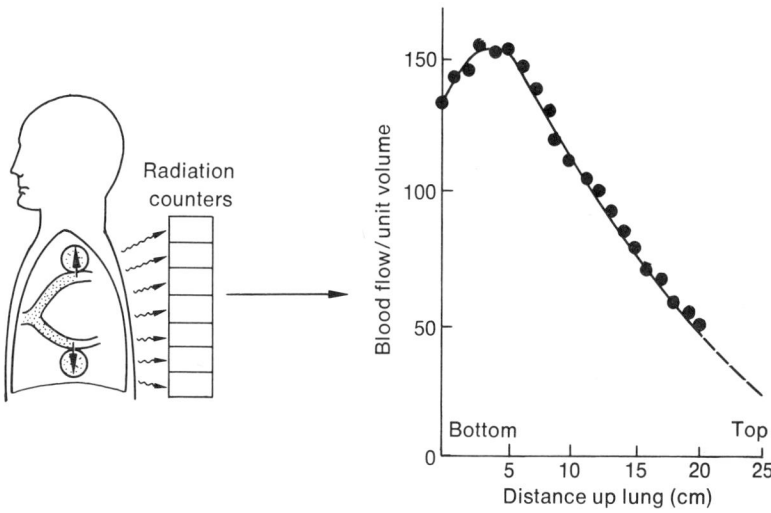

FIGURE 4-17. Measurement of the distribution of blood flow in the upright human lung using radioactive xenon. The dissolved xenon is evolved into alveolar gas in the pulmonary capillaries. The units of blood flow are such that if flow were uniform, all values would be 100. Note the small flow at the apex. (From J. M. B. Hughes, J. B. Glazier, J. E. Maloney, and J. B. West. *Respir. Physiol.*, **4**: 58, 1968.)

near the bottom of the upright lung and gradually decrease as we go toward the top. However, blood flow decreases more rapidly than ventilation so that the $\dot{V}_e/\dot{Q}_e$ ratio rises rapidly as the top of the lung is approached (Figure 4-18). This means that the equilibrium gas tensions differ from the top to the bottom in a manner that is summarized in Figure 4-19. Thus, at the top, the local $\dot{V}_e/\dot{Q}_e$ ratio is 3.3 and the equilibrium gas tensions are $P_{e_{CO_2}} = 28$ and $P_{e_{O_2}} = 132$. At the bottom, the corresponding values are $\dot{V}_e/\dot{Q}_e = 0.63$, $P_{e_{CO_2}} = 42$, and $P_{e_{O_2}} = 89$. Despite these rather marked differences, weighted averages for blood and gas phases reveal a resulting mixed $P_e - P_a$ gradient of less than 1 mm Hg for P_{CO_2} but about 4 mm Hg for P_{O_2}. Thus our practice of using $P_{a_{CO_2}}$ to estimate $P_{e_{CO_2}}$ (see pp. 56–57) is still reasonably accurate in a normal subject despite the presence of some $\dot{V}_e/\dot{Q}_e$ nonuniformity.

THREE-COMPARTMENT DESCRIPTION OF $\dot{V}_e/\dot{Q}_e$ NONUNIFORMITY. Instead of trying to quantitate the continuous distribution of $\dot{V}_e/\dot{Q}_e$ ratios that actually exist in the effective gas exchanger (e.g., Figures 4-15 and 4-18), it is much simpler for practical purposes to use an equivalent three-compartment model comprising (1) an "ideal" uniform effective exchanger whose $\dot{V}_e/\dot{Q}_e$ ratio is consistent with overall

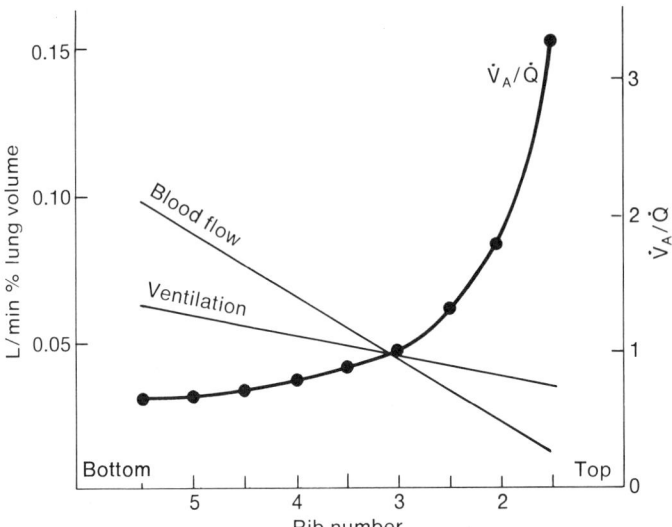

FIGURE 4-18. Distribution of ventilation and blood flow down the upright lung. Note that the ventilation-perfusion ratio decreases down the lung. (From J. B. West. *Ventilation/Bloodflow and Gas Exchange.* Oxford: Blackwell Scientific Publications, Ltd., 1970.)

gas exchange, (2) an alveolar shunt compartment with $\dot{V}_e/\dot{Q}_e = 0$, and (3) an alveolar dead space with $\dot{V}_e/\dot{Q}_e = \infty$. This procedure, introduced by Riley and Cournand in 1949 (*11*), has really been the basis for our overall diagram of the exchange apparatus shown in Figure 4-2. We can illustrate the general principles involved with the aid of Figure 4-20, a simplified modification of Figure 4-14.

The composition of the "ideal" compartment, i, is located at the intersection of the blood and gas R-lines corresponding to the overall gas exchange ratio. We then assume that any departure of the actual arterial point from point i is due to an alveolar shunt, i.e., to a mixing of ideal blood with mixed venous blood. The magnitude of the shunt determines the movement of the arterial point, a, along the blood R line from i toward $\bar{V}$. Note that because the blood R line is nearly horizontal over much of its range, $P_{a_{CO_2}}$ remains very close to $P^i_{CO_2}$ unless the shunt becomes extremely large. In practice we assume that $P^i_{CO_2}$ is equal to $P_{a_{CO_2}}$, as we have noted before, and then we can calculate the corresponding $P^i_{O_2}$ from an appropriate modification of equation (26):

$$P^i_{O_2} = P_{i_{O_2}} - \frac{1}{R}P_{a_{CO_2}} \tag{40}$$

Thus we really need not use the graphical method to obtain the ideal

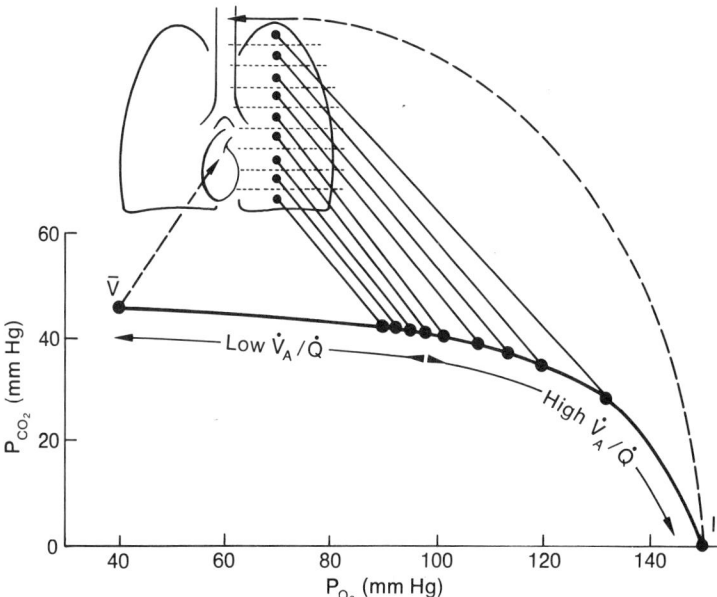

FIGURE 4-19. Result of combining the pattern of ventilation-perfusion ratio inequality with the effects of this on gas exchange. Note that the high ventilation-perfusion ratio at the apex results in a high P_{O_2} and low P_{CO_2} there. The opposite is seen at the base. (From J. B. West. *Ventilation/Bloodflow and Gas Exchange*. Oxford: Blackwell Scientific Publications, Ltd., 1970.)

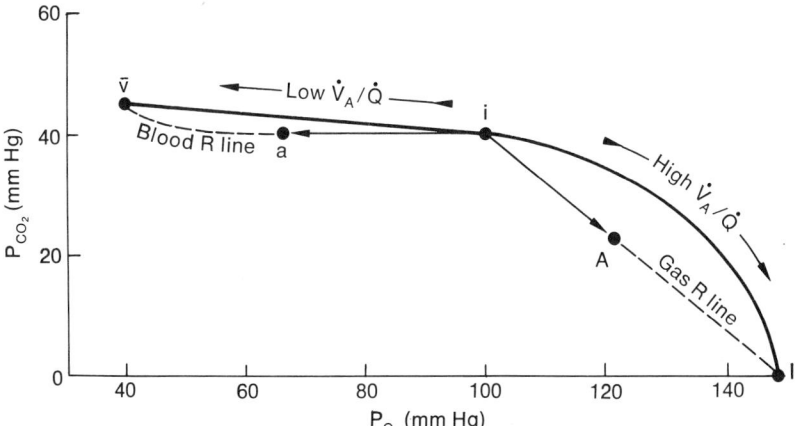

FIGURE 4-20. O_2-CO_2 diagram showing the ideal point, i, that is the hypothetical composition of alveolar gas and end-capillary blood when no ventilation-perfusion inequality is present. As inequality develops, the arterial a and alveolar A points diverge along their respective R (respiratory exchange ratio) lines. The mixed alveolar-arterial P_{O_2} difference is the horizontal distance between the points. (From J. B. West. *Respiratory Physiology*. Baltimore: The Williams & Wilkins Company, © 1974.)

point. Note from the graph, however, that the flatness of the blood R-line, which is responsible for the minimal departure of P_{aCO_2} from $P^i_{CO_2}$, has just the opposite significance for P_{aO_2}, which rapidly moves away from $P^i_{O_2}$ even with a very small shunt. We have noted this before, and this is why we cannot obtain $P^i_{O_2}$ directly from P_{aO_2} even in normal people but must instead calculate it from P_{aCO_2} using equation (40).

Finally, we assume that any departure of the mixed alveolar point, A, from i is due to an alveolar dead space, i.e., to a mixing of ideal gas with inspired gas. The magnitude of the dead space determines the movement of the alveolar point along the gas R line from i toward I.

RECENT DEVELOPMENTS IN MEASURING $\dot{V}/\dot{Q}$ DISTRIBUTIONS

Although the three-compartment analysis just described is both practical to carry out and clinically useful, efforts to obtain a more detailed resolution of the $\dot{V}/\dot{Q}$ distribution within the active exchanger persist. A recent technique developed by Wagner appears promising for this purpose. It is based on intravenous infusion of six inert, soluble gases and the measurement of their expired and arterial gas concentrations. Estimates of the distribution of ventilation-perfusion ratio are made by applying a simple model of gas exchange in the steady state. Let us briefly review the basis of their approach.

If an inert gas is dissolved in saline and injected continuously into a peripheral vein at a constant rate until a steady state is reached, the lungs will expire the same quantity of gas per minute. This mass balance is described by

gas flux from blood = expired gas rate

or

$$Q_i(C_{\bar{v}} - C_{ec_i}) = \dot{V}_{A_i} F_{A_i} \qquad (41)$$

where Q_i = blood flow rate
$C_{\bar{v}}$ = mixed venous inert gas concentration
C_{ec_i} = end capillary inert gas concentration
$\dot{V}_{A_i}$ = alveolar ventilation
F_{A_i} = alveolar fraction of inert gas

and i refers to the ith lung exchanger unit shown schematically in Figure 4-21. This model corresponds to one of many parallel units that are perfused by mixed venous blood and ventilated by inspired gas. Mixed venous blood and inspired gas are assumed to be the same for

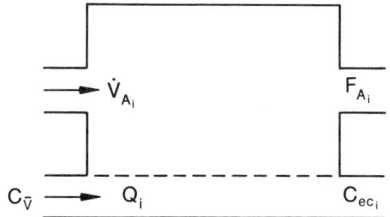

FIGURE 4-21.   Inert gas exchange model of ith parallel lung unit.

all units with inspired test gas concentrations assumed to be zero. Alveolar fraction can be related to alveolar partial pressure as

$$F_A = \frac{P_A}{P_B - P_{H_2O}} \tag{42}$$

where P_A = alveolar partial pressure
P_B = barometric pressure
P_{H_2O} = vapor pressure of water

Also, gas contents can be related to partial pressures as

$$C_{\bar{V}} = SP_{\bar{V}} \tag{43}$$

and

$$C_{ec} = SP_{ec} \tag{44}$$

where S = inert gas solubility
$P_{\bar{V}}$ = mixed venous partial pressure
P_{ec} = end capillary partial pressure

Substituting these relationships into equation (41) yields

$$Q_i S(P_{\bar{V}} - P_{ec_i}) = \dot{V}_{A_i} \frac{P_{A_i}}{P_B - P_{H_2O}} \tag{45}$$

If we assume that alveolar and end capillary partial pressures are equal ($P_{ec_i} = P_{A_i}$), and define a blood-gas partition coefficient, λ, as

$$\lambda = S(P_B - P_{H_2O}) \tag{46}$$

equation (45) can be written as

$$\frac{P_{A_i}}{P_{\bar{V}}} = \frac{\lambda}{(\dot{V}_{A_i}/Q_i) + \lambda} \tag{47}$$

Since we have assumed a model with N parallel pathways, mixed expired (assuming zero dead space) and arterial partial pressures are described for gas by

$$P_A \sum_{i=1}^{N} \dot{V}_{A_i} = \sum_{i=1}^{N} P_{A_i} \dot{V}_{A_i} \qquad (48)$$

and for blood by

$$P_a \sum_{i=1}^{N} Q_i = \sum_{i=1}^{N} P_{A_i} Q_i \qquad (49)$$

where P_A = mixed alveolar partial pressure
P_a = arterial partial pressure

By substituting equation (47) in (48) and (49) and rearranging, we get finally:

$$\frac{P_A}{P_{\bar{V}}} = \frac{\sum_{i=1}^{N} \frac{\lambda \dot{V}_{A_i}}{(\dot{V}_{A_i}/Q_i) + \lambda}}{\sum_{i=1}^{N} \dot{V}_{A_i}} \qquad (50)$$

and

$$\frac{P_a}{P_{\bar{V}}} = \frac{\sum_{i=1}^{N} \frac{\lambda Q_i}{(\dot{V}_{A_i}/Q_i) + \lambda}}{\sum_{i=1}^{N} Q_i} \qquad (51)$$

Since $\sum_{i=1}^{N} \dot{V}_{A_i} = \dot{V}_A$ (total alveolar ventilation) and $\sum_{i=1}^{N} Q_i = Q$ (cardiac output), the measurements of these two parameters as well as the partial pressures of mixed alveolar air (P_A), mixed venous blood ($P_{\bar{V}}$), and arterial blood (P_a) for various inert gases (different values of λ) permit Q_i to be calculated as a function of $\dot{V}_{A_i}/Q_i$ from equation (51) and $\dot{V}_{A_i}$ as a function of $\dot{V}_{A_i}/Q_i$ from equation (50). Obviously, there are limitations on the number of such pairs possible, due to the limited number of gases used. If equations (50) and (51) are applied directly, the use of six gases permits at most six ventilations and flows to be uniquely determined at six selected values of ventilation-perfusion ratios. In practice, numerical smoothing methods are used to estimate continuous distribution curves. However, the resolution of these curves is similarly restricted by the number of gases used. Despite this limitation, additional diagnostic information over and above that possible with three-compartment analysis appears to be possible using this approach.

Disturbances of the Pulmonary Gas Exchanger

It is convenient to summarize the properties of the pulmonary gas exchanger by examining the general classes of abnormalities that may arise in disease and the measurements that reveal their presence. We can list four such general abnormalities:

1. Inefficient gas delivery.
2. Inefficient blood delivery.
3. Diffusion block.
4. Inefficient gas-blood matching ($\dot{V}/\dot{Q}$ maldistribution).

The first of these is revealed by a low effective fraction, eF, and thus by a low expired-arterial P_{CO_2} ratio, $P_{E_{CO_2}}/P_{a_{CO_2}}$. Alternatively, we could call this a high total physiologic dead space, or $(1 - eF)$. We recall that a low eF can result from a low alveolar fraction (AF = $P_{E_{CO_2}}/P_{A_{CO_2}}$), a low effective alveolar fraction (eAF = $P_{A_{CO_2}}/P_{a_{CO_2}}$), or both. A low alveolar fraction (or increased physiologic conductive dead space) can result from an increase in conductive airway volume, as in bronchiectasis, a decrease in tidal volume as in the tachypnea of pneumonia, or from both. A low effective alveolar fraction (or increased alveolar dead space) can arise from a pulmonary embolus that blocks blood flow to a ventilated alveolar area of the lung, or from a $\dot{V}/\dot{Q}$ maldistribution with or without a true alveolar dead space component.

Inefficient blood delivery can be caused by a true anatomic shunt bypassing the lungs as in congenital heart disease, or by continued perfusion of nonventilated alveoli (i.e., an alveolar shunt), which may occur in local airway obstruction and atelectasis. The increased venous admixture from either cause is revealed by an increase in the $P_{A_{O_2}} - P_{a_{O_2}}$ gradient. Such an increase can also be produced by a true diffusion block such as may arise in pulmonary fibrosis. In the latter case, there should also be a low diffusion capacity, D_{O_2}. Moreover, breathing a high oxygen mixture will generally reduce a gradient caused by diffusion block but will not affect one caused by venous admixture.

Finally, $\dot{V}/\dot{Q}$ maldistributions probably occur in a variety of pulmonary diseases but are particularly characteristic of chronic obstructive lung disease ("COLD," or chronic bronchitis and emphysema), and the adult respiratory distress syndrome (ARDS or shock lung). Such maldistributions are revealed by a simultaneous increase in apparent alveolar dead space (i.e., a low $P_{A_{CO_2}}/P_{a_{CO_2}}$) and venous admixture or apparent alveolar shunt (i.e., an increased $P_{A_{O_2}} - P_{e_{O_2}}$

gradient). This is now thought to be the major cause of arterial hypoxemia in COLD.

The disturbances just described and the measurements that reveal their presence are summarized in Table 4-5.

TABLE 4-5

	eF	AF	eAF	$P_{AO_2}-P_{aO_2}$	D_{O_2}	Sh
1. Inefficient gas delivery	−					
a. Conductive	−	−				
(1) Structural (bronchiectasis)	−	−				
(2) Functional (tachypnea)	−	−				
b. Alveolar	−		−			
2. Inefficient blood delivery				+		+
3. Diffusion block				+	−	+
4. Gas-blood mismatch ($\dot{V}/\dot{Q}$ maldistribution)		−		+		+

References

1. Bouhnys, A. Distribution of inspired gas in the lungs. In: *Handbook of Physiology*, Section 3, *Respiration*, Vol. 1. Edited by W. O. Fenn and Herman Rahn. Washington, D. C.: American Physiological Society, 1964, pp. 715–733.
2. Forster, R. E. Rate of reaction of CO_2 with human hemoglobin. In: CO_2-*Chemical, Biochemical and Physiological Aspects*. Edited by R. E. Forster, J. T. Edsall, A. B. Otis, and F. J. W. Roughton. Washington, D.C.: National Aeronautics and Space Administration, 1969, pp. 55–59.
3. Forster, R. E., and E. D. Crandall. Time course of exchanges between red cells and extracellular fluid during CO_2 uptake. *J. Appl. Physiol.* 38: 710–718, 1975.
4. Hill, E. P., G. G. Power, and L. D. Longo. Kinetics of O_2 and CO_2 exchange. In: *Lung Biology in Health and Disease* (Executive Editor, Claude Lenfant), Vol. 3: *Bioengineering Aspects of the Lung*. Edited by John B. West. New York: Marcel Dekker, Inc., 1977, pp. 459–514.
5. Hlastala, M. P. A model of fluctuating alveolar gas exchange during the respiratory cycle. *Respir. Physiol.* 15: 214–232, 1972.
6. Kelman, G. R. Computer program for the production of O_2-CO_2 diagrams. *Respir. Physiol.* 4: 260–269, 1968.
7. Olszowka, A. J., and L. E. Farhi. A digital computer program for constructing ventilation perfusion lines. *J. Appl. Physiol.* 26: 141–146, 1969.
8. Rahn, H. A concept of mean alveolar air and the ventilation-bloodflow relationships during pulmonary gas exchange. *Am. J. Physiol.* 158: 21–30, 1949.

9. Rahn, H., and L. E. Farhi. Ventilation, perfusion, and gas exchange, the $\dot{V}_A/\dot{Q}$ concept. In: *Handbook of Physiology*, Section 3, *Respiration*, Vol. 1. Edited by W. O. Fenn and Herman Rahn. Washington, D. C.: American Physiological Society, 1964, pp. 735–766.
10. Rahn, H., and W. O. Fenn. *A Graphical Analysis of the Respiratory Gas Exchange*. Washington, D. C.: American Physiological Society, 1955.
11. Riley, R. L., and A. Cournand. "Ideal" alveolar air and the analysis of ventilation-perfusion relationships in the lungs. *J. Appl. Physiol.* 1: 825–847, 1949.
12. Roughton, F. J. W. Transport of oxygen and carbon dioxide. In: *Handbook of Physiology*, Section 3, *Respiration*, Vol. 1. Edited by W. O. Fenn and Herman Rahn. Washington, D. C.: American Physiological Society, 1964, pp. 767–825.
13. Wagner, P. D., H. A. Saltzman, and J. B. West. Measurement of continuous distributions of ventilation-perfusion ratios: Theory. *J. Appl. Physiol.* 36: 484–599, 1974.
14. Wagner, P. D., and J. B. West. Effects of diffusion impairment on O_2 and CO_2 time course in pulmonary capillaries. *J. Appl. Physiol.* 33: 62–71, 1972.
15. Weibel, E. R. *Morphometry of the Human Lung*. New York: Academic Press, Inc., 1963.
16. Weibel, E. R., and J. Gil. Structure-function relationships at the alveolar level. In: *Lung Biology in Health and Disease* (Executive Editor, Claude Lenfant), Vol. 3: *Bioengineering Aspects of the Lung*. Edited by John B. West. New York: Marcel Dekker, Inc., 1977, pp. 1–82.
17. West, J. B. *Respiratory Physiology*. Baltimore: The Williams & Wilkins Company, 1974.
18. West, J. B. *Ventilation/Blood Flow and Gas Exchange*, 3rd ed. Oxford: R. H. Blackwell, Ltd., 1976.
19. West, J. B., and P. D. Wagner. Pulmonary gas exchange. In: *Lung Biology in Health and Disease* (Executive Editor, Claude Lenfant), Vol. 3: *Bioengineering Aspects of the Lung*. Edited by John B. West. New York: Marcel Dekker, Inc., 1977, pp. 361–457.

CHAPTER 5

Tissue Gas Exchange

JUST AS THE ALVEOLI are ventilated by air, the tissues are "ventilated" by blood to provide oxygen, remove carbon dioxide, and equilibrate nitrogen. This gas exchange function of the tissues requires the coordination of the cardiovascular and respiratory systems. In this chapter, the nature of this coordination and the major driving forces of diffusion and perfusion are presented.

Diffusion of Oxygen

A. Krogh (1) was the first to advance the hypothesis that diffusion alone is sufficient to explain oxygen exchange from blood to tissue. His work was based on the idealized capillary-tissue model shown in Figure 5-1. This model assumes a homogeneous tissue space with each capillary supplying a cylindrical tissue volume. Thus the entire metabolizing tissue mass is conceptually divided into many parallel identical units. For a capillary of length ℓ, the rate at which oxygen is used by the tissue located between r and R is

$$(\pi R^2 \ell - \pi r^2 \ell) \frac{\dot{V}_{O_2}}{V} \quad (1)$$

where $\dot{V}_{O_2}$ = total tissue oxygen consumption and V = total tissue volume. The quantity $\pi R^2 \ell - \pi r^2 \ell$ is the tissue volume located

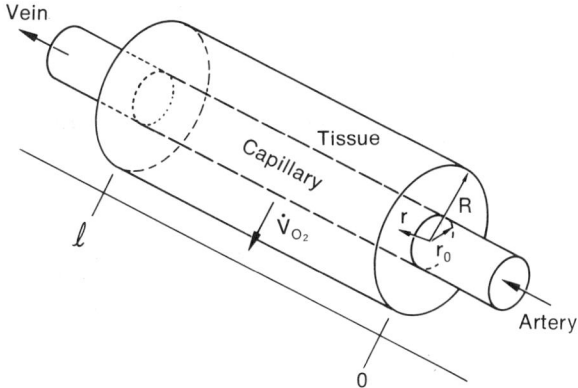

FIGURE 5-1. Krogh capillary-tissue model.

between r and R. The rate at which oxygen diffuses through the cylindrical surface at radius r, dQ/dt, is

$$\frac{dQ}{dt} = -2\pi r \ell \alpha D \frac{dP_{T(O_2)}}{dr} \quad (2)$$

where D = diffusion coefficient (cm^2/sec)
   α = solubility coefficient (ml gas/ml fluid · mm Hg)
   $2\pi r \ell$ = surface area at radius r
   $dP_{T(O_2)}/dr$ = oxygen tension gradient at radius r

The product αD is often referred to as Krogh's diffusion coefficient.

In the steady state, if no other source of oxygen supply is available, the rate of utilization will match the rate of diffusion yielding

$$(\pi R^2 \ell - \pi r^2 \ell)\frac{\dot{V}_{O_2}}{V} = -2\pi r \ell \alpha D \frac{dP_{T(O_2)}}{dr} \quad (3)$$

Equation (3) can be considered to be a quantitative statement of Krogh's hypothesis. Thus comparisons of predictions of equation (3) with experimental data constitute a test of this hypothesis. Solution of equation (3) is easily accomplished by separation of variables yielding the following equation defining the capillary-tissue oxygen tension gradient:

$$P_{T(O_2)}(r_0) - P_{T(O_2)}(r) = \frac{\dot{V}_{O_2}}{2\alpha DV}\left[R^2 \ln \frac{r}{r_0} - \frac{(r^2 - r_0^2)}{2}\right] \quad (4)$$

Krogh reasoned that by substituting r = R in the above equation the tension difference necessary to supply the entire tissue by diffusion is obtained. If this difference is found to be smaller than the venous blood tension, then every point in the tissue space can be supplied by diffusion alone. Using guinea pig muscles, Krogh estimated the various parameter values of equation (4) and found that venous blood tension was high enough to conclude that diffusion alone could explain muscle-tissue oxygen supply.

In recent years, there have been a number of attempts (*2, 3, 4*) to use the above "Krogh cylinder" model to make theoretical estimates of the oxygen gradient occurring in various tissues. Based on this approach, Thews (*2*) has predicted an oxygen tension gradient for human brain tissue of 17 mm Hg from cylinder center to periphery at the venous end of the capillaries. In a similar manner, estimates have also been made of time-varying oxygen gradients in human myocardial tissue (*2*). In general, such predictions suggest that a significant difference in oxygen tension exists between various parts of the tissue. However, experimental support of these predictions is not conclusive. Thus it can only be said that such tension gradients lie within the realm of possibility.

Diffusion of Carbon Dioxide

Since tissue O_2 exchange can be adequately explained by passive diffusion, it follows *a fortiori* that CO_2 elimination can be fully explained by diffusion also. This is because the diffusion coefficients for both gases are similar and the solubility coefficient of CO_2 is about 20 times that of O_2. According to equation (4), this means that the required capillary-tissue tension gradient for CO_2 is only $\frac{1}{20}$ that for O_2. Therefore, if the O_2 tension gradient is 17 mm Hg at the venous end as mentioned above, then the corresponding CO_2 tension gradient is only 0.75 mm Hg. Clearly, the movement of CO_2 within tissue by diffusion is so efficient that no significant gradient is possible within various parts of the tissue. Although the chemical reactions of CO_2 in blood, as noted in Chapter 4, may not normally reach equilibrium in the time taken for a red cell to traverse a capillary so that P_{CO_2} and pH changes may continue, this does not appear to be rate limiting for overall O_2 or CO_2 exchange. The major rate limiting factor is blood flow (perfusion).

We shall next consider the effects of perfusion, but prior to this we wish to add these words of caution: Although it is tempting to conclude that diffusion alone is responsible for both oxygen and carbon dioxide exchange in tissue, this conclusion cannot be made on the basis of the above arguments, which only show that diffusion *is capable* of providing sufficient exchange. Whether or not this passive physical mechanism is solely responsible for tissue gas exchange is still open to question as indicated by certain observations to the contrary (4, 5). However, it is certainly true that diffusion is the dominant factor involved in oxygen and carbon dioxide exchange.

Perfusion Limited Exchange

If tissue does not have a significant tension gradient within it and both chemical and diffusion equilibria are reached essentially instantaneously, then it will behave primarily as a uniform storage volume for the gas in question. Since these assumptions are normally valid for CO_2, let us consider such a model. The conceptual diagram of the model is shown in Figure 5-2. The following equation describes the

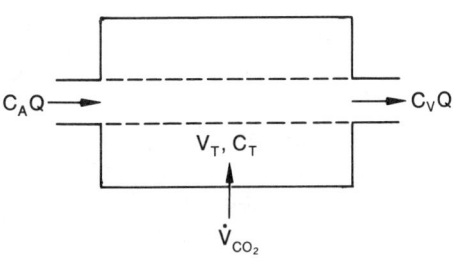

FIGURE 5-2.   Model of perfusion limited exchange.

CO_2 mass balance indicated in the figure:

$$\frac{dC_T}{dt} V_T = C_A Q + \dot{V}_{CO_2} - C_V Q \qquad (5)$$

or in words,

rate of accumulation = rate of entry + rate of production

−rate of departure,

where C_A = arterial blood CO_2 content (liter CO_2/liter blood)
 C_T = tissue CO_2 content
 C_V = venous blood CO_2 content
 $\dot{V}_{CO_2}$ = rate of tissue production of CO_2
 Q = tissue blood flow
Since we have assumed an adequate diffusion,

$$P_{V_{CO_2}} = P_{T_{CO_2}} \qquad (6)$$

The dissociation curves (C vs. P_{CO_2}) for blood and tissue are nonlinear functions. However, over a reasonable physiologic range, a linear approximation can be made of the form (6)

$$C = a + bP_{CO_2} \qquad (7)$$

Strictly speaking, the linear approximation for tissue dissociation is slightly different than for blood (7), and probably differs for different tissues, but we shall assume equality for simplicity. This results in the following form of equation (5):

$$\frac{V_T}{Q}\frac{dP_{TCO_2}}{dt} = P_{ACO_2} - P_{TCO_2} + \frac{\dot{V}_{CO_2}}{bQ} \qquad (8)$$

In the steady state, $dP_T/dt = 0$ and the CO_2 tension of tissue becomes

$$P_{TCO_2} = P_{ACO_2} + \frac{\dot{V}_{CO_2}}{bQ} \qquad (9)$$

From equation (9), it is evident that by varying Q any tension higher than P_{ACO_2} can be achieved. The quantity V_T/Q in equation (8) is the time constant of tissue exchange. For a step change in P_{ACO_2}, the time constant indicates the time following the step initiation at which the response is 63% completed. For a normal man, the total tissue volume, V_T = 40 liters, and cardiac output, Q = 6 L/min, which leads to

$$\frac{V_T}{Q} = 6.6 \text{ min} \qquad (10)$$

The magnitude of this time constant is what largely determines the length of time required for equilibrium to be reached in CO_2 stores following disturbances in respiration. As apparent from equation (8), a transient alteration in Q (cardiac output) will also cause a CO_2 stores disturbance. Such transients in gas stores are important in connection with chemical regulation of respiration as discussed in Chapter 7.

Inert Gas Exchange

Chemically inert gases such as nitrogen or anesthetics move from blood to tissue by diffusion alone. Since there is no net production or utilization of these gases within tissue, no steady-state gradient of tensions within tissue is possible. Thus the dynamics of inert gas exchange is of greater concern. Interest in this area has been greatly stimulated by the importance that such exchange plays in decompression sickness.

Since the time of P. Bert (8) it has been known that gas bubbles resulting from the release of dissolved tissue gas (primarily nitrogen) are the basic cause of the symptoms of decompression sickness. The primary disturbance here is sudden alteration from high to low barometric pressure, and this is a common occupational hazard for divers, caisson workers, pilots, and personnel involved in hyperbaric oxygenation therapy. At sea level, a normal man has about 1 liter of N_2 dissolved in blood and tissue. If barometric pressure is raised by 1 atm, the weight of dissolved N_2 doubles but the volume of N_2 (expressed at ambient P) remains the same. This follows from the ideal gas law, which states that

$$PV = nRT \qquad (11)$$

Pressure increases by a factor of two, which one would normally expect to lead to a corresponding halving of volume, but n doubles by Henry's law and V remains constant, since T is also constant at body temperature. When this quantity of gas is returned to sea level, the 1 liter of gas expands to 2 liters, which is 1 liter more than blood and tissue can hold at sea level pressure. This is the origin of the gas bubbles that lead to the symptoms of decompression sickness. These can include pain in the extremities (bends), numbness in the joints, and even unconsciousness (9). The only way to avoid these symptoms is to decompress at a rate slow enough to allow the respiratory system to eliminate this excess N_2. The most effective decompression technique to be developed is "stage decompression."

In 1908, Haldane (10) made a brilliant observation that revolutionized decompression methods. Haldane found that decompression from 2 to 1 atm could be accomplished in man without any precautions. No matter what the duration of the exposure to 2 atm, rapid decompression to 1 atm never resulted in any symptoms of decompression sickness. Haldane then reasoned that the same volume of dissolved gas would be liberated by expansion any time the absolute pressure is halved. Thus if it is safe to decompress rapidly from 2 to 1 atm, it would be equally safe to decompress from 4 to 2 or 8 to 4 atm. The basis for this statement is shown in Table 5-1. Listed in that table are the volumes of N_2 in the body (assumed to be 1 liter at sea level) at ambient pressure and compressed or expanded to other pressures. One liter of N_2 is liberated when pressure is changed from 2 to 1, 4 to 2, or 8 to 4 atm. Haldane verified the correctness of this reasoning using animals initially and finally man. Thus the initial step in stage decompression is a rapid decompression to half of the original ambient

TABLE 5-1
N_2 Volume Changes due to Pressure.
Equivalent volumes correspond to constant number of molecules

P (atm)	Volume at Ambient P (liter)	Equiv. Volume at 1 atm (liter)	Equiv. Volume at 2 atm (liter)	Equiv. Volume at 4 atm (liter)
1	1	1	0.5	0.25
2	1	2	1	0.5
4	1	4	2	1

pressure. This is followed by decompression in fixed pressure steps that are taken each time the N_2 partial pressure has dropped an amount corresponding to twice the size of the pressure step. This procedure is best illustrated by an example. However, first we need to consider the dynamics of tissue N_2.

To describe the dynamics of tissue N_2, we shall make the same perfusion-limited assumptions as for CO_2 exchange. This results in the model shown in Figure 5-3. The following mass balance equation applies for N_2 exchange:

$$\frac{V_T \alpha_T}{Q \alpha_B} \frac{dP_{T_{N_2}}}{dt} = P_{A_{N_2}} - P_{T_{N_2}} \tag{12}$$

where α_T = tissue N_2 solubility and α_B = blood N_2 solubility. The time constant of N_2 exchange, $V_T \alpha_T / Q \alpha_B$, is thus a direct function of tissue solubility and inverse function of flow. The solubility of N_2 in fat is about five times that in blood or water, so organs with high fat contents (bone marrow, spinal cord, adipose tissue) are expected to have long desaturation times. For a step change in $P_{A_{N_2}}$ caused by decompression, tissue such as bone marrow requires approximately 2 hr to be 63% desaturated (9). Let us now consider the application of stage decompression based on a desaturation time constant of 108 min (10).

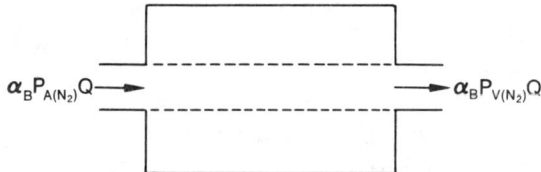

FIGURE 5-3. Perfusion-limited model of tissue N_2 dynamics.

As an example, consider the case of a dive to a depth of 213 ft, where the period of exposure is sufficient to insure complete N_2 saturation at that depth. Since the depth corresponds to 213 + 33 = 246 ft of water in absolute pressure, the first step would be to reduce this pressure to half or 123 ft H_2O. From here ascents will be made in increments of 10 ft. The first increment is made when the N_2 partial pressure corresponds to air at 226 ft H_2O (decrease of 20 ft H_2O). The time required for a decrease of ΔPN_2 partial pressure when the step change in pressure is P is

$$t = -\tau \ln\left(1 - \frac{\Delta P}{P}\right) \qquad (13)$$

where $\tau = N_2$ exchange time constant. For the first level, assuming $\tau = 108$ min the time required is

$$t_1 = -108 \ln\left(1 - \frac{20}{123}\right) = 19.2 \text{ min}$$

The new depth is then 113 ft H_2O and the next increment is made when the N_2 partial pressure corresponds to air at 206 ft H_2O. The time required for this decrease is

$$t_2 = -108 \ln\left(1 - \frac{20}{113}\right) = 21.0 \text{ min}$$

These depth increments progress in this way until the surface is reached. Table 5-2 shows the length of time required at each depth for complete stage decompression.

TABLE 5-2

Depth Pressure (ft H_2O)	Time at Level (min)
246	Saturation
123	19.2
113	21.0
103	23.3
93	26.2
83	29.8
73	34.6
63	41.2
53	51.2
43	67.6
33 (surface)	—

In the case of dives of shorter duration, the procedure for decompression would be analogous except that the dive duration would be used to estimate the initial level of tissue N_2 partial pressure. Standard tables for decompression based on this general approach are available (*11*).

References

1. Bailey, H. R. Oxygen exchange between capillary and tissue: Some equations describing countercurrent and nonlinear transport. In: *Physical Bases of Circulatory Transport: Regulation and Exchange.* Philadelphia: W. B. Saunders Company, 1967, pp. 353–366.
2. Behnke, A. R., Jr., and E. H. Lanphier. Underwater physiology. In: *Handbook of Physiology,* Section 3, *Respiration,* Vol. 2. Edited by W. O. Fenn and H. Rahn. Washington: American Physiological Society, 1965, pp. 1159–1193.
3. Bert, P. *Barometric Pressure: Researches in Experimental Physiology.* (English translation.) Columbus, Ohio: College Book Company, 1943.
4. Boycott, A. E., G. C. C. Damant, and J. S. Haldane. The prevention of compressed air illness. *J. Hyg. (Camb.)* 8: 342–443, 1908.
5. Defares, J. G., H. E. Derksen, and J. W. Duyff. Cerebral bloodflow in the regulation of respiration. *Acta Physiol. Pharmacol. Neerlandica,* 9: 327–360, 1960.
6. Grodins, F. S., J. S. Gray, K. R. Schroeder, A. L. Norins, and R. W. Jones. Respiratory responses to CO_2 inhalation: A theoretical study of a nonlinear biological regulator. *J. Appl. Physiol.* 7: 283–308, 1954.
7. Gurtner, G. H., S. H. Song, and L. E. Farhi. Alveolar to mixed venous P_{CO_2} difference under conditions of no gas exchange. *Respir. Physiol.* 7: 173–187, 1969.
8. Krogh, A. *The Anatomy and Physiology of Capillaries.* New York: Hafner Publishing Co., Inc., 1959.
9. Otis, A. B. Some simple models for the diffusion of oxygen from blood to tissue. In: *Physical Bases of Circulatory Transport: Regulation and Exchange.* Philadelphia: W. B. Saunders Company, 1967, pp. 367–370.
10. Thews, G. Gaseous diffusion in the lungs and tissues. In: *Physical Bases of Circulatory Transport: Regulation and Exchange.* Philadelphia: W. B. Saunders Company, 1967, pp. 327–341.
11. Workman, R. D. Standard decompression procedures and their modification in preventing the bends. *Ann. N.Y. Acad. Sci.* 117: 834–842, 1965.

CHAPTER

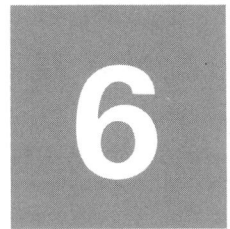

Blood Buffers and Acid-Base Balance

Introduction

IN CHAPTER 1, we noted the central role of the concept of homeostasis or regulation in physiology. One of the important regulated variables of the internal environment is its hydrogen ion concentration, $[H^+]$. Thus the $[H^+]$ of arterial blood is normally kept very close to 38.9 nM/L corresponding to a pH of 7.41. This normal value is protected by a combination of passive (chemical) and active (physiologic) buffering. The respiratory system and the kidney are most important in the latter. To appreciate how they work, we must first review some basic concepts of passive (chemical) buffers.

A chemical buffer consists of a mixture of a weak acid and its salt. If we consider the weak acid, carbonic acid, we can write its primary ionization as follows:

$$\underset{\text{Weak acid}}{H_2CO_3} \rightleftarrows \underset{\text{Conjugate base}}{HCO_3^-} + \underset{\text{Hydrogen ion}}{H^+} \tag{1}$$

and define the equilibrium (ionization, dissociation) constant, K, according to the mass action law:

$$\frac{[H^+][HCO_3^-]}{[H_2CO_3]} = K \tag{2}$$

and rearranging:

$$[H^+] = K\frac{[H_2CO_3]}{[HCO_3^-]} \tag{3}$$

By definition, a weak acid has a very small dissociation constant so that most of it exists in solution as the undissociated acid with only a tiny fraction in the form of conjugate base and hydrogen ions.

On the other hand, the salt, $NaHCO_3$, is almost completely dissociated in solution so that very nearly all of it is present as Na^+ and HCO_3^-. If then we have a buffer solution in the form of a mixture of both H_2CO_3 and $NaHCO_3$, we can make certain approximations in equation (3) by considering that the concentration of undissociated acid, $[H_2CO_3]$, is essentially equal to the total acid concentration, and that the concentration of conjugate base, $[HCO_3^-]$, is essentially equal to the total salt concentration, $[NaHCO_3]$. We can then write equation (3) in several equivalent forms as follows:

$$[H^+] = K'\frac{[H_2CO_3]}{[NaHCO_3]} = K'\frac{[acid]}{[salt]} = K'\frac{[HA]}{[BA]}$$

$$= K'\frac{[acid]}{[conjugate\ base]} = K'\frac{[HA]}{[A^-]} \tag{4}$$

The "prime" on the K indicates that it now includes the approximations noted above, and the last four forms of the equation simply generalize it to include any buffer mixture, where HA and BA represent any weak acid and its salt. Equation (4) is known as the Henderson equation after Lawrence J. Henderson (1878–1942), professor of physiological chemistry at Harvard, whose classic book published in 1928 (2) described blood as a physicochemical system.

Equation (4) was modified by K. A. Hasselbalch to yield pH rather than $[H^+]$:

$$pH = -\log[H^+] = -\log K' - \log\frac{[acid]}{[salt]} \tag{5}$$

or

$$pH = pK' + \log\frac{[salt]}{[acid]} \tag{6}$$

Equation (6) is the Henderson-Hasselbalch equation, which is generally useful in defining the relative salt and acid concentrations required to produce a buffer mixture of a given pH. Note that when the ratio of [salt]/[acid] = 1, pH = pK'.

We can now make clear how a chemical buffer can minimize changes in pH on the addition of either a strong acid, Ha, or a strong base, BOH. If we add Ha, then the H^+ contributed by the highly dissociated acid is tied up by the conjugate base, A^-, in the form of the weak acid, HA. If we add BOH, then the OH^- contributed by the highly dissociated base is tied up by the H^+ from HA in the form of water. In the former case, the ratio of [salt]/[acid] in equation (6) decreases and pH falls somewhat; in the latter, this ratio increases and the pH rises somewhat, but in both the changes in pH are much less than they would be if Ha or BOH were added to pure water. In both cases also, although the [salt]/[acid] ratio changes, the sum of the two buffer components remains constant. This is the essence of passive chemical buffering.

Active or physiologic buffering implies that some physiologic control mechanism can alter the total quantity of either the acid or salt of the buffer mixture by retaining it in or excreting it from the body. For example, if a strong acid were injected into the blood, it would not only be passively buffered by the $BHCO_3/H_2CO_3$ system, as described above, but the respiratory system would immediately excrete increased amounts of H_2CO_3 via the lungs (i.e., as CO_2) to prevent an excessive fall in the $[BHCO_3]/[H_2CO_3]$ ratio and thus in pH. We shall see how this works in detail in what follows.

Blood Buffers

Blood is a multiple buffer system, but the most important components for our purposes are the bicarbonate and protein buffers, the latter comprising both plasma proteins and the hemoglobin of the red blood cells:

$$\frac{BHCO_3}{H_2CO_3} \quad \frac{BP}{HP} \quad \frac{BHb}{HHb} \quad \frac{BHbO_2}{HHbO_2}$$

The $BHCO_3/H_2CO_3$ buffer is most important in buffering against strong acids whereas the protein buffers are most important in buffering carbonic acid itself and thus play an important role in normal CO_2 transport by the blood. For the former we can write

$$Ha + BHCO_3 \rightleftarrows Ba + H_2CO_3 \tag{7}$$

and for the latter

$$H_2CO_3 + BP' \rightleftarrows BHCO_3 + HP' \tag{8}$$

where P' now represents all of the protein components.

How can we best describe this multiple buffer system in a way that is both rigorously quantitative and yet relatively simple and convenient? When we consider the complications involved, it at first seems like a hopeless task. Thus blood is a two-phase system, and although some of the buffer components occur in both phases (i.e., $BHCO_3/H_2CO_3$), others are limited to plasma (BP/HP) or to red cells (BHb/HHb; $BHbO_2/HHbO_2$). Moreover, the "B" in plasma is mainly sodium and that in red cells is mainly potassium, and the two do not exchange freely across the red cell membrane, a problem the blood solves by the *Hamburger* or *chloride shift* (*1*). Finally, HHb is a weaker acid (and thus a better buffer against H_2CO_3) than $HHbO_2$ (the *Haldane effect*). Despite all these complications, however, it turns out that we can achieve a simple graphic description of the system.

Let us begin by going back to the Henderson-Hasselbalch equation as it applies to a simple $BHCO_3/H_2CO_3$ buffer system:

$$pH = pK' + \log \frac{[BHCO_3]}{[H_2CO_3]} \tag{9}$$

Although this equation cannot be applied directly to the two-phase system of whole blood, it does apply to plasma alone. If we always use "true plasma," i.e., plasma that has come to acid-base equilibrium with its red cells before it is separated for analysis, then the behavior of this plasma will reflect the activity of all of the blood buffers, cellular as well as extracellular. For application to plasma we can rewrite equation (9) by noting that $[H_2CO_3]$ is directly proportional to P_{CO_2} (Henry's law, Chapter 2), and if $[BHCO_3]$ is expressed in mM/L and P_{CO_2} in mm Hg, we have

$$pH = 6.10 + \log \frac{[BHCO_3]}{0.0301 P_{CO_2}} \tag{10}$$

Now equation (10) defines simultaneously compatible values for the three variables, $[BHCO_3]$, P_{CO_2}, and pH. For graphic representation we can regard one of these as a parameter defining a family of curves relating the other two. The choice is arbitrary and none is without some disadvantage. However, a popular plot is shown in Figure 6-1 in which P_{CO_2} is taken as the parameter for a family of curves relating $[BHCO_3]$ to pH (*1, 14*). For each fixed value of P_{CO_2} (e.g., the normal 40 mm Hg), the curve is an exponential function:

$$[BHCO_3] = A \cdot 10^{pH-6.10} \tag{11}$$

where the value of A depends upon the number assigned to P_{CO_2}. The

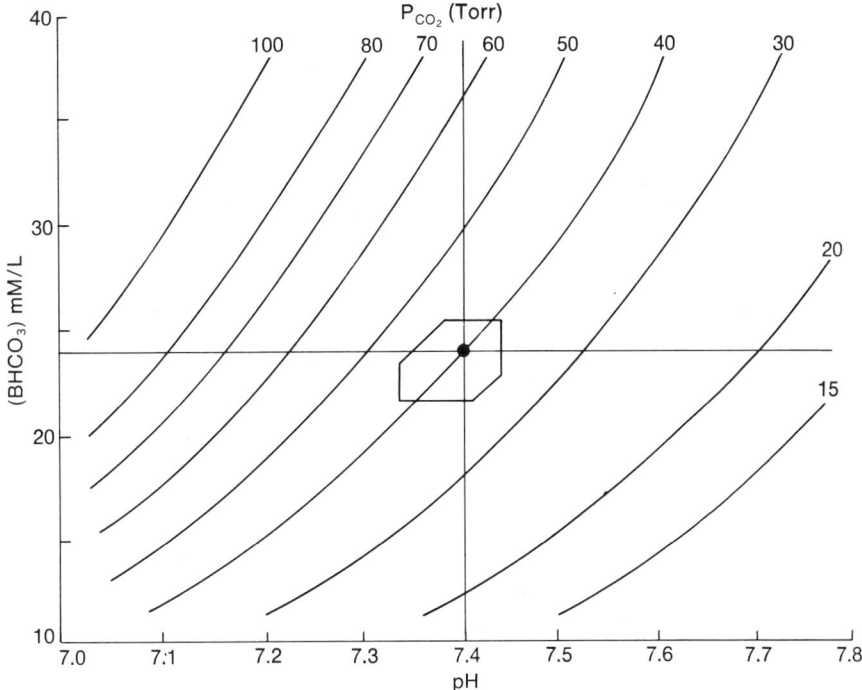

FIGURE 6-1. The [BHCO₃]-pH diagram for blood plasma.

average normal arterial point is shown on the $P_{CO_2} = 40$ isobar at pH = 7.40 and [BHCO₃] = 24.0 with a range of normal variation indicated around it.

Titration of Blood—Passive Chemical Buffering

TITRATION WITH CARBONIC ACID

We recall that the BP′/HP′ system is the primary buffer against H_2CO_3 [see equation (8)]. Hence, if we titrate blood with carbonic acid *in vitro* by equilibrating it with gas mixtures of known P_{CO_2}, the resulting curve for true plasma, when plotted on our [BHCO₃]-pH diagram, will define the passive buffer properties of the nonbicarbonate (i.e., the protein) buffers of blood. One of the advantages of this form of plot is that the CO_2 titration (or "absorption") curve turns out to be linear over the physiologic pH range, and its slope, $\Delta[BHCO_3]/\Delta pH$, directly defines the "buffer capacity" of the protein buffer systems. Since hemoglobin is the most important of these protein buffers, it is not surprising that the buffer slope is a function of the hemoglobin concentration:

$$-\frac{\Delta[BHCO_3]}{\Delta pH} = 8.2 + 1.56[Hb] \tag{12}$$

where [Hb] is total hemoglobin concentration in g/100 ml. We also recall that the degree of oxygenation of hemoglobin influences its buffer properties, but it turns out that this factor only affects the position of the titration curve and not the slope, e.g., the curve for fully reduced blood is parallel to but about 3 mM/L [BHCO$_3$] above that for fully oxygenated blood. We have plotted these curves for true plasma from oxygenated and reduced normal blood ([Hb] = 15 g %) in Figure 6-2.

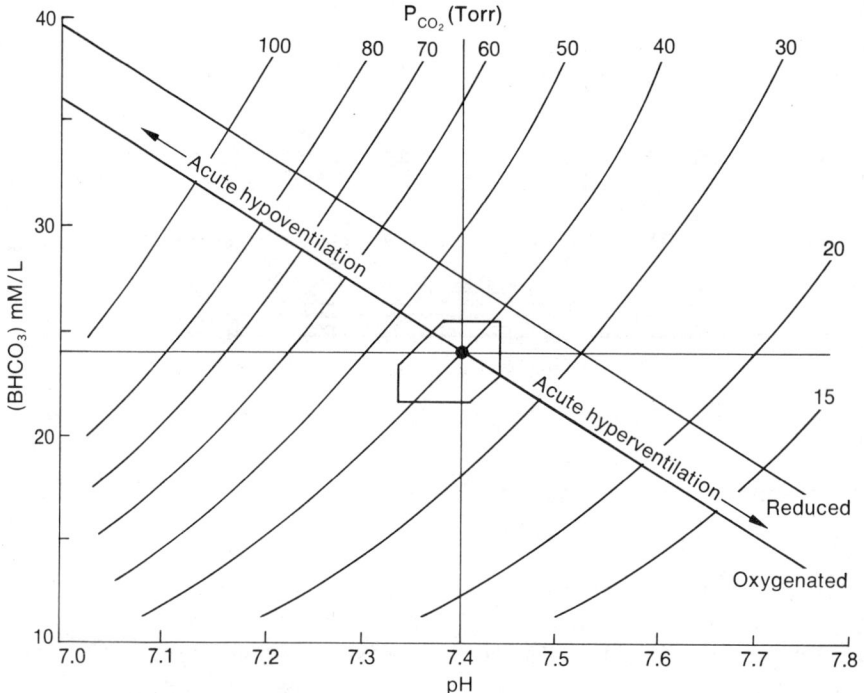

FIGURE 6-2. The BP′/HP′ buffer curves for true plasma.

Now the curve from oxygenated blood not only describes how arterial (i.e., essentially fully oxygenated) blood would behave if titrated with H$_2$CO$_3$ *in vitro*, but *in vivo* as well, provided no physiologic compensation or "active buffering" occurs. The latter in this case would involve increased excretion or retention of $BHCO_3$ by the kidney and this is a relatively slow process requiring days to weeks. Hence the behavior of arterial blood during acute hyperventilation or hypoventilation, that amounts to *in vivo* titration of blood with H_2CO_3 since P_{aCO_2} is primarily determined by ventilation (Chapter 4), follows this passive nonbicarbonate buffer line. The operating point moves to the left along this line during hypoventilation and to the right during hyperventilation as indicated in Figure 6-2.

Finally, as we shall see below, changes in the vertical position of this true plasma nonbicarbonate buffer curve reflect the addition or removal of fixed strong acid.

TITRATION WITH Ha

The $BHCO_3/H_2CO_3$ system is the major passive buffer for strong fixed acid (e.g., HCl or "Ha") [equation (7)] although it is clear from equation (8) that some of the H_2CO_3 generated in the process will in turn be buffered by the BP'/HP' system. Hence when we titrate blood with Ha, the resulting titration curve will in general reflect the buffer contributions of both systems. If we arrange to carry out this titration at constant P_{CO_2} (which we can do by adding Ha to blood that is equilibrated with a gas mixture of fixed P_{CO_2}), the titration curve will follow the corresponding P_{CO_2} isobar on our $[BHCO_3]$-pH diagram. This would be true for a pure bicarbonate buffer as well as for the multiple buffer system of blood. However, in the former, if we added 5 mM/L of Ha, then $[BHCO_3]$ would also fall 5 mM/L to point A on the $P_{CO_2} = 40$ isobar in Figure 6-3, whereas in blood, the fall in $[BHCO_3]$ would be less than this (i.e., to point B) because some of the H_2CO_3 formed by reaction (7) is converted back to $BHCO_3$ by the BP' system [equation (8)]. If we draw a BP'/HP' buffer line through B parallel to the normal line and "back titrate" the system along this line by lowering P_{CO_2} until we reach point C at normal pH = 7.4, we shall restore the BP'/HP' system to its original condition, i.e., at constant pH, all Ha is buffered by the $BHCO_3/H_2CO_3$ system and none by the protein systems. Thus given any point such as A or B on our $[BHCO_3]$-pH diagram, we can determine how much strong acid excess or deficit is present by drawing a BP'/HP' buffer line through this point and extrapolating it to pH 7.4.

It turns out that the $\Delta[BHCO_3]_{7.4}$ so obtained does not quite represent the true acid excess or deficit because there is a slight difference between the true plasma and whole blood buffer slopes that is a function of hemoglobin concentration. This is incorporated in a correction factor introduced by Siggaard-Anderson (8) to calculate the *base excess of blood* (BE_b) from the $\Delta[BHCO_3]_{7.40}$ of true plasma

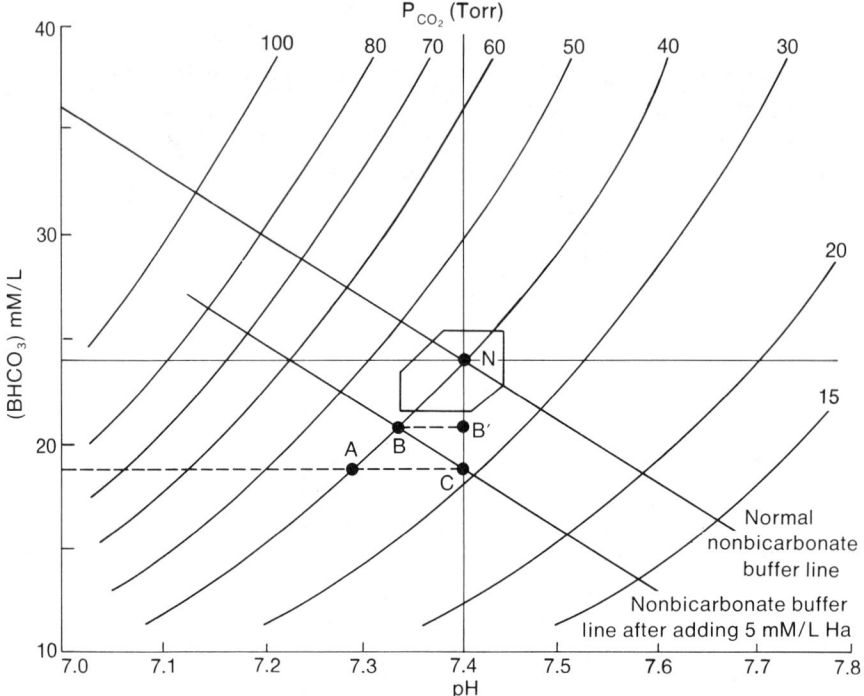

FIGURE 6-3. Titration of blood with Ha. $NC = \Delta[BHCO_3]_{7.40} = -\text{total Ha}$; NB' = portion of Ha buffered by bicarbonate during iso-P_{CO_2} titration; $B'C$ = portion of Ha buffered by protein during iso-P_{CO_2} titration; and A = iso-P_{CO_2} titration end point for pure bicarbonate buffer system.

obtained as described above:

$$BE_b = (1 - 0.0125[Hb])\Delta[BHCO_3]_{7.40} \qquad (13)$$

where (Hb) is hemoglobin concentration in g/100 ml and BE_b is expressed in mEq/L. For a normal [Hb] = 15 gm/100 ml, this becomes

$$BE_b = 0.81\Delta[BHCO_3]_{7.40} \qquad (14)$$

The following empirical formula can be used to estimate the base excess in the entire extracellular space (8):

$$BE_{ECS} = 0.3 BE_b \times W \qquad (15)$$

where W is body weight in kilograms. This formula has been used as a guide in estimating the amount of acid or base that can safely be used to correct any deficit or excess in patients. Extracellular space BE is used rather than whole body BE in an attempt to prevent transient overcorrection of the extracellular space.

Although the base excess concept appears useful as a clinical guide, the application of formulas such as equation (15) must be approached with caution. One must constantly be aware of the fact that the state of blood is determined by the combined action of blood buffers, lung, and kidney. Thus the fact that the base excess parameter is high or low does not necessarily indicate the need for corrective measures. The potential clinical difficulties that arise if one does not appreciate this limitation are discussed by Schwartz and Relman (7). We shall consider some of them when we discuss active or physiologic buffering and introduce some basic concepts of disturbances in acid-base balance.

Active or Physiologic Buffering—Disturbances in Acid-Base Balance and Their Compensation

We can most simply define a disturbance in acid-base balance as a condition characterized by an abnormal pattern of P_{aCO_2}, $[BHCO_3]_P$, $[BHCO_3]_{7.40}$, and pH_a. The first two of these quantities are almost always involved; the last two may or may not be. We can best describe these disturbances in terms of their primary cause and the nature of their physiologic compensation.

METABOLIC DISTURBANCES AND THEIR RESPIRATORY COMPENSATION

A metabolic disturbance in acid-base balance is caused by the addition of a strong acid or strong base to the blood. Historically, the metabolic acidoses associated with severe diabetes (abnormal production of ketone acids) or with nephritis (failure to excrete fixed acid products of normal metabolism) were the first to be recognized and studied. From the standpoint of the blood buffer systems, the primary disturbance is a shift in the level of the nonbicarbonate buffer curve that we can characterize by the value of $[BHCO_3]_{7.40}$, the *standard bicarbonate content* (Figure 6-4).

The course that the operating point will follow in moving from one of these lines to another depends upon active respiratory compensation. Since P_{aCO_2} is determined by ventilation, we would follow the $P_{CO_2} = 40$ isobar if ventilation remained constant at its normal level, moving up the isobar in metabolic alkalosis and down it in metabolic acidosis. However, we hinted in Chapter 1, and shall discover in detail

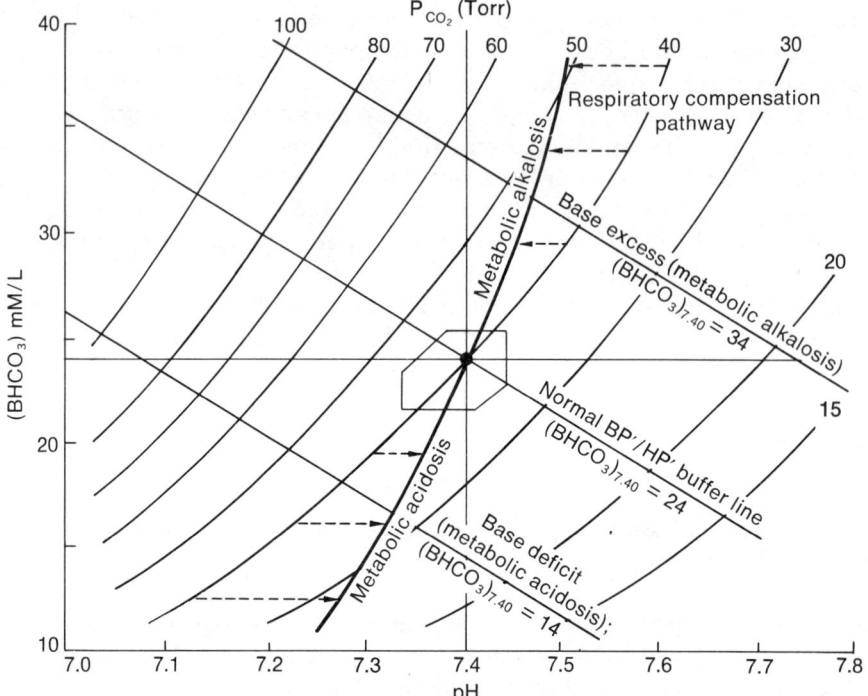

FIGURE 6-4. Metabolic disturbances and their respiratory compensation. The BP'/HP' *buffer lines* for normal, base excess, and base deficit. The *Respiratory (active) compensation pathway* based on Gray's equation. Horizontal dashed arrows between this pathway and $P_{CO_2} = 40$ isobar show the degree of pH correction achieved by respiratory compensation.

in Chapter 7, that the changes in pH so induced will alter ventilation in such a way as partially to correct this pH change. Since P_{aCO_2} varies inversely with $\dot{V}_A$, we can calculate this correction from a modification of Gray's equation [equation (4), Chapter 7]:

$$\frac{\dot{V}_A}{\dot{V}_{A_0}} = \frac{P_{aCO_2}(\text{normal})}{P_{aCO_2}(\text{disturbance})} = 0.22[H^+]_a + 0.262 P_{aCO_2} - 18 \quad (16)$$

The respiratory compensation pathway defined by equation (16) is also shown in Figure 6-4, and the degree of pH correction that it achieves is indicated by the horizontal dashed arrows. Note that this respiratory compensation is rapid but never complete, i.e., some pH error always remains.

RESPIRATORY DISTURBANCES AND THEIR RENAL COMPENSATION

A respiratory disturbance in acid-base balance is caused by the addition to, or subtraction of, carbonic acid from the blood. Since $[H_2CO_3]_a$ is directly proportional to P_{aCO_2} and the latter is a function of ventilation, such disturbances are (with the exception of CO_2 inhalation) due to effective hyperventilation or hypoventilation. We have already noted that active compensation for a respiratory disturbance involves excretion or retention of $BHCO_3$ by the kidneys, an action that alters $[BHCO_3]_{7.40}$. However, we also noted that renal compensation is very slow so that in acute respiratory disturbances, $[BHCO_3]_{7.40}$ remains normal and our operating point moves to the left or right along the normal BP'/HP' buffer line (Figure 6-2). But how does our operating point move as renal compensation begins?

We have shown some representative pathways in Figure 6-5. In acute hyperventilation (e.g., exposure to high altitude), we move along the normal BP' buffer line from point N to point A; $[BHCO_3]_{7.40}$ is normal at this stage and point N represents a completely uncompensated metabolic alkalosis. What renal compensation does is to produce a metabolic acidosis (i.e., a reduction in $[BHCO_3]_{7.40}$) to compensate for the respiratory alkalosis. As this develops, we move from point A to point D along what is really a *respiratory compensation line* similar to, but displaced to the right from, the normal pathway shown in Figure 6-4 and repeated in Figure 6-5 running through point N. Note that although renal compensation is slow, it is eventually complete; i.e., the pH returns to normal. In acute respiratory acidosis, we move from point N to B, and then as renal compensation begins, we go slowly along another "respiratory compensation pathway" from B to C.

Some Principles of Diagnosis

Interpreted in isolation, blood acid–base data can be treacherous, particularly if incomplete. For example, the low P_{CO_2} and $[BHCO_3]$ characteristic of point A are compatible with either a respiratory alkalosis (which it is) or a metabolic acidosis (which it is not). If we thought it were the latter, we might treat the patient with $NaHCO_3$ which would be disastrous! The determination of pH and $[BHCO_3]_{7.40}$ would resolve the problem. A thorough understanding of the principles described in this chapter together with the clinical history, physical, and laboratory findings will usually produce a correct interpretation of the significance of any given point on our acid-base

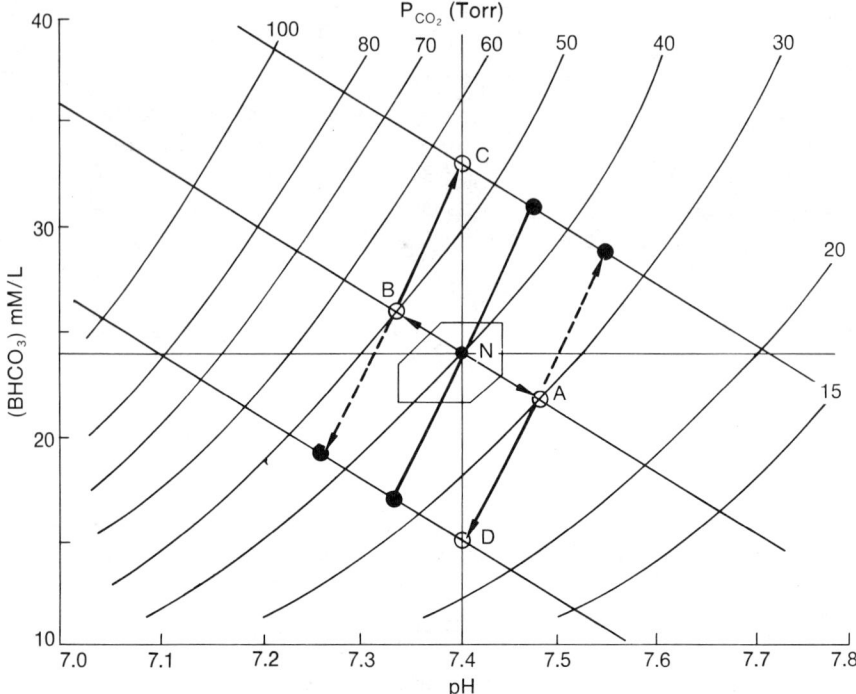

FIGURE 6-5. Respiratory disturbances and their renal compensation.
N–A–D = primary respiratory alkalosis and its renal compensation
    A = acute respiratory alkalosis
    D = complete renal compensation
N–B–C = primary respiratory acidosis and its renal compensation
    B = acute respiratory acidosis
    C = complete renal compensation

diagram. We need to consider the probable primary cause (respiratory or metabolic), the presence and degree of physiologic compensation, and the acute or chronic nature of the disturbance.

References

1. Davenport, H. W. *The ABC of Acid-Base Chemistry*. Chicago: University of Chicago Press, 1969.
2. Henderson, L. J. *Blood, A Study in General Physiology*. New Haven, Conn.: Yale University Press, 1928.
3. Hills, A. G. *Acid-Base Balance Chemistry, Physiology, and Pathophysiology*. Baltimore: The Williams & Wilkins Company, 1973.

4. Leusen, I. Regulation of cerebrospinal fluid composition with reference to breathing. *Physiol. Rev.* **52**: 1–56, 1972.
5. Peters, J. P., H. A. Bulger, and A. J. Eisenman. Studies of the CO_2 absorption curve of human blood. IV. The relation of the hemoglobin content of blood to the form of the CO_2 absorption curve. *J. Biol. Chem.* **58**: 747–768, 1923–1924.
6. Peters, J. P., and D. D. Van Slyke. *Quantitative Clinical Chemistry*, Vol. 1, *Interpretations*. Baltimore: The Williams & Wilkins Company, 1932, pp. 868–1018.
7. Schwartz, W. B., and A. S. Relman. A critique of the parameters used in the evaluation of acid-base disorders. *N. Engl. J. Med.* **268**: 1382–1387, 1963.
8. Siggaard-Andersen, O. *The Acid-Base Status of the Blood*. Baltimore: The Williams & Wilkins Company, 1964.
9. Van Slyke, D. D. On the measurement of buffer values and on the relationship of buffer value to the dissociation constant of the buffer and the concentration and reaction of the buffer solution. *J. Biol. Chem.* **52**: 525–570, 1922.
10. Van Slyke, D. D., A. B. Hastings, M. Heidelbeiger, and J. M. Neill. Studies of gas and electrolyte equilibria in blood. III. The alkali-binding and buffer values of oxyhemoglobin and reduced hemoglobin. *J. Biol. Chem.* **54**: 481–506, 1922.
11. Van Slyke, D. D., and J. Sendroy, Jr. Studies of gas and electrolyte equilibria in blood. XV. Line charts for graphic calculations by the Henderson-Hasselbalch equation and for calculating plasma CO_2 content from whole blood content. *J. Biol. Chem.* **79**: 781–798, 1928.
12. Waddell, W. J., and R. G. Bates. Intracellular pH. *Physiol. Rev.* **49**: 285–329, 1969.
13. Winters, R. W., K. Engel, and R. B. Dell. *Acid-Base Physiology in Medicine. A Self-Instruction Program*. Westlake, Ohio: The London Co., 1967.
14. Woodbury, J. W. Regulation of pH. In: *Physiology and Biophysics*, 20th ed., Vol. 2. Edited by T. C. Ruch and H. D. Patton. Philadelphia: W. B. Saunders Company, 1974, pp. 480–524.

CHAPTER

7

Control of Pulmonary Ventilation

Introduction

IN THE FIRST CHAPTER of this book we said that a real understanding of the overall behavior of the respiratory system required knowledge of both its individual unit processes and of their interactions. We have now described many of the former in some detail and it now remains to examine the latter. We also hinted in Chapter 1 that the most interesting type of interaction was negative feedback, a characteristic feature of both man-made physical, and naturally occurring biologic, control systems. Finally, we said that in this context we could regard the respiratory system as a "metabolic servomechanism" designed to match pulmonary and metabolic gas exchange rates by appropriate manipulation of pulmonary ventilation. It is this theme that we shall develop in the present chapter.

What do we mean by a control system, or a servomechanism, or negative feedback? It turns out that it is hard to talk about control without lapsing into the language of teleology. Thus a man-made physical control system does not exist until the engineer designs and builds it to accomplish a particular purpose or goal. Biologic control systems preexist in nature, but we have no way of knowing what "purpose" or "goal," if any, their designer intended for them. Nevertheless, it is both convenient and fruitful to describe such systems "as if" they were "purposefully designed" or "goal directed" without

CONTROL OF PULMONARY VENTILATION   109

worrying about the broader philosophical implications that others may read into such descriptions.

In this spirit we can now describe the general pattern and purpose of feedback control systems, whether man-made or biologic. In so doing, we shall make use of the *block diagram* notation, a very convenient descriptive tool in systems analysis that we used without elaboration in Figure 1-2. In this notation, each "unit process" is represented by a block having an input and an output (Figure 7-1). The

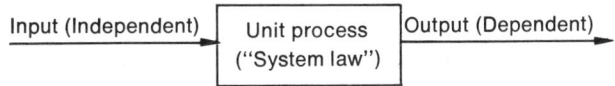

FIGURE 7-1.   Block diagram of unit process.

output (or dependent variable) depends upon the input (or independent variable) according to a definite "system law," which may be expressed verbally, graphically, or mathematically. Interactions between these "unit processes" can then be easily expressed by appropriate connections between the unit blocks. In this notation we can recognize two major blocks or unit processes in every feedback control system: (1) a controlled system (or plant), and (2) a controlling system (or controller); these are arranged in a "closed-loop" or "feedback" pattern (Figure 7-2). The goal or purpose of such an arrangement

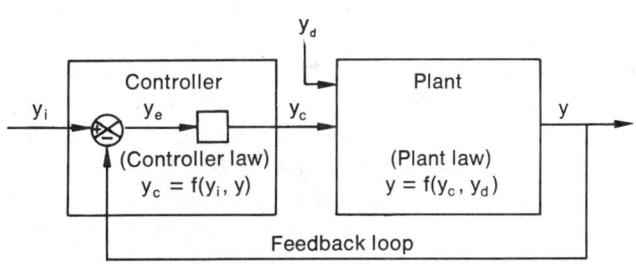

FIGURE 7-2.   Block diagram of feedback control system.

is to keep the output of the plant (the regulated variable, y) equal or at least close to some desired value (y_i) despite disturbances (y_d) that tend to upset this correspondence. To accomplish this, information about the value of y is "fed back" to the controller where it is compared to y_i to generate an *error signal*,

$$y_e \equiv y_i - y$$

The controller then translates y_e into a *controlling signal*, y_c, which causes the plant to change its output in a direction appropriate to reduce y_e. Thus any deviation of y from y_i is "automatically" corrected either completely (integral controller),

$$y_c = K_I \int y_e \, dt$$

or partially (proportional controller),

$$y_c = K_P y_e$$

If the system is primarily designed to keep y close to a constant y_i (*set point*), it is called a regulator; if to "track" a y_i that changes appreciably with time, it is called a servomechanism. A familiar example of the former is a room temperature control system, of the latter an antiaircraft fire control system.

In man-made physical control systems all of the elements illustrated in Figure 7-2 and described above can be explicitly identified. Thus we all know how to adjust the "set point" of our house thermostat, and the subtraction of y from y_i to generate y_e is performed by a specific physical device, a *comparator*, that we can identify. Incidentally, it is this subtraction (or sign reversal around the loop) that makes the feedback system "negative" and insures that the corrections will be made in the appropriate direction. In biologic control systems, however, it is generally impossible to identify an independent set point or a comparator. We can recognize an implicit set point as the normal operating point collectively determined by all of the system parameters, but we do not know "where it is" or "how to adjust it independently," if indeed these are meaningful questions. Similarly, whereas we can identify the sign reversal around the loop, which is the *sine qua non* of negative feedback, it is not performed by a simple comparator but rather is an input-output property of some particular component of either the plant or controller. Thus, for example, increased pulmonary ventilation reduces $P_{a_{CO_2}}$; reduced $P_{a_{O_2}}$ increases carotid body receptor discharge, etc., etc.

With this background, let us now attempt to describe the control of pulmonary ventilation. We shall begin with the basic respiratory chemostat first proposed in quantitative form by J. S. Gray in 1945.

Basic Steady-State Respiratory Chemostat

The observation that arterial hypercapnia, acidemia, and hypoxemia increase pulmonary ventilation, whereas voluntary hyperventilation produces arterial hypocapnia, alkalemia, and hyperoxemia, sets the stage for the concept of a closed-loop respiratory chemostat. If we take the system to be a regulator designed to keep arterial P_{CO_2}, $[H^+]$, and P_{O_2} nearly constant in the presence of certain particular disturbances, we can first describe its operation in qualitative terms. Thus if we breathe 5% CO_2 in air, P_{aCO_2} and $[H^+]_a$ rise. Both changes stimulate ventilation, and the increased ventilation in turn lowers P_{aCO_2} and $[H^+]_a$ back toward normal values. If we inject a strong acid into the blood, $[H^+]_a$ rises and this stimulates ventilation. The increased ventilation decreases P_{aCO_2} below normal and thus drops $[H^+]_a$ back toward normal. Finally, if we breathe a gas mixture deficient in oxygen, P_{aO_2} falls and this fall stimulates ventilation. The increase in ventilation raises P_{aO_2} back toward normal but also produces hypocapnia and alkalemia.

From this qualitative behavior it is clear that we are dealing with a feedback regulator that is concerned with at least three regulated variables, P_{aCO_2}, $[H^+]_a$, and P_{aO_2}. It is also clear that the system shows some "steady-state error" in the presence of the above disturbances; i.e., the regulated variables do not return completely to their normal values. Finally, it appears that in some instances, e.g., hypoxia, a response designed to correct the primary disturbance may cause errors in other regulated quantities.

Let us draw a block diagram of this control system similar to, but not identical with, Figure 7-2. The differences incorporate the points mentioned previously, i.e., no explicit set points or comparators, as well as the fact that we must deal with three regulated variables instead of only one. The choice of which processes to include in the plant block and which to assign to the controller is often somewhat arbitrary and frequently a matter of convenience. The choice we have made here is the one originally made by Gray and will serve to start us off. In it, many of the details of unit processes that we have considered in previous chapters (e.g., ventilatory mechanics, gas and blood distribution, etc.) do not appear explicitly at all, and are thus implicitly concealed either within the plant or controller blocks. This concealment really involves the assumption that these details are normal and invariant, and since we cannot measure many of them conveniently anyway, this approach more clearly reveals the essence of the "respiratory chemostat" in normal man.

As shown in Figure 7-3, the input to the plant is taken as alveolar ventilation, $\dot{V}_A$, and the outputs as arterial CO_2 tension, P_{aCO_2}, oxygen tension, P_{aO_2}, and hydrogen ion concentration, $[H^+]_a$. Thus the plant contents must include most of the pulmonary gas exchanger and the blood buffer system. To obtain the *plant law*, i.e., the dependence of P_{aCO_2}, P_{aO_2}, and $[H^+]_a$ on $\dot{V}_A$, Gray made many simplifying

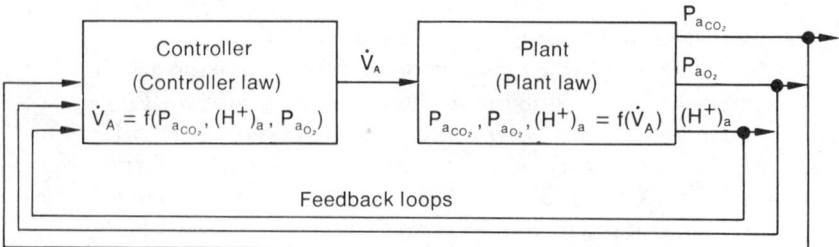

FIGURE 7-3. Block diagram of basic respiratory chemostat.

assumptions, e.g., steady-state; equality of $\dot{V}_A$ and $\dot{V}_e$; equality of alveolar, effective, and arterial gas tensions; and known values of $\dot{V}_{O_2}$ and $\dot{V}_{CO_2}$. He could thus avoid treating the exchange process in detail and obtain the output gas tensions, P_{aCO_2} and P_{aO_2}, from a simple mass-balance accounting for the gas phase alone as explained in Chapter 4 (see pp. 58–60). If the minor effect of R's less than 1 on this accounting is neglected, the process becomes particularly simple. Thus the alveolar (and hence the effective and arterial) CO_2 tension is simply the sum of the tracheal CO_2 tension, P_{iCO_2} (normally zero), and the increment produced by adding the metabolic CO_2 production, $\dot{V}_{CO_2}$, to the alveolar ventilation, $\dot{V}_A$ [cf. equations (23) and (24), Chapter 4]:

$$P_{aCO_2} = P_{ACO_2} = P_{iCO_2} + \frac{863 \dot{V}_{CO_2}}{\dot{V}_A} \tag{1}$$

and similarly for oxygen:

$$P_{aO_2} = P_{AO_2} = P_{iO_2} - \frac{863 \dot{V}_{O_2}}{\dot{V}_A} \tag{2}$$

where 863 is the constant incorporating barometric pressure and reconciling STPD (for $\dot{V}_{CO_2}$) and BTPS (for $\dot{V}_A$) units of volume, as noted in Chapter 4. These two plant equations are thus the essence of simplicity, depend only upon gas phase mass balance relations, and are perfectly satisfactory as long as we deal with normal subjects in the steady state.

We have yet to obtain a third plant law, i.e., the dependence of $[H^+]_a$ on $\dot{V}_A$. We do this indirectly using equations (1) and (2), the oxygen dissociation curve described in Chapter 4, and the properties of the blood buffer system described in Chapter 6. It should be clear in principle that if we know P_{aCO_2}, P_{aO_2} (and thus O_2 saturation), total Hb, and $[BHCO_3]_{7.4}$, we can obtain pH_a (and thus $[H^+]_a$) either from a graphic solution such as given in Figures 6-2 to 6-5 or from the following rather formidable-looking equation in which $[H^+]_a$ is a rather awkward implicit function of these input variables:

$$P_{a_{CO_2}} = \frac{[H^+]_a}{53.3}\{(16 + 2.30_{2_{150}})(\log[H^+]_a - 1.59)$$

$$+ [BHCO_3]_{7.4} + 0.375(O_{2_{150}} - O_2)\}, \quad (3)$$

where $O_{2_{150}}$ is oxygen capacity (dependent on total Hb) and O_2 is oxygen content (dependent on both total Hb and P_{O_2}). In Figure 7-4 we have drawn an explicit block for this blood-buffer component of the plant for further clarification.

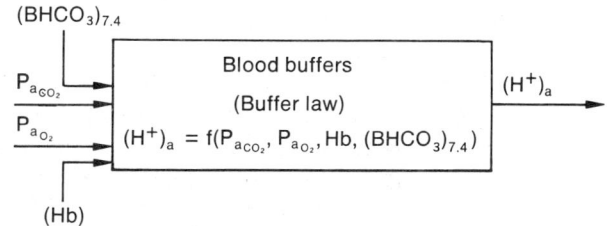

FIGURE 7-4. Block diagram of blood buffer system.

Finally, let us note that all three "plant laws" are based on physical and chemical principles that would hold just as well *in vitro* as *in vivo*. This is in marked contrast to the *controller law* to which we now turn our attention.

Let us note first that the output of the "controller" is taken as alveolar ventilation, $\dot{V}_A$, and the inputs as $P_{a_{CO_2}}$, $P_{a_{O_2}}$, and $(H^+)_a$, and that the "controller law" must define the dependence of the former on the latter. There are obviously a great many unit processes in between, some of which we have not even described morphologically, let alone functionally. Thus, concealed within this block are all of the central and peripheral sensory mechanisms that respond to these chemical agents, the respiratory centers that process this sensory information, the motor fibers to the respiratory muscles, the entire ventilatory apparatus described in Chapter 3, and the exchanger apparatus described in Chapter 4. Gray's description of the controller law was a purely empirical one based upon observed ventilatory responses to CO_2 inhalation, metabolic acidosis and alkalosis, and arterial hypoxemia. The simplest equation compatible with all of these observed responses was

$$\dot{V}_A = \dot{V}_{A_0}\{0.22[H^+]_a + 0.262 P_{a_{CO_2}} + (105 \times 10^{-0.038 P_{a_{O_2}}}) - 18\} \quad (4)$$

where $\dot{V}_{A_0}$ is normal resting $\dot{V}_A$ at sea level breathing air. Gray's conceptual description of this equation at the time it was formulated was that each of the three arterial chemical agents, P_{aCO_2}, $[H^+]_a$, and P_{aO_2}, exerted an independent stimulating effect on ventilation, and that the actual ventilation was the sum of the partial effects of all three. This was taken to be a revolutionary concept at the time when the most burning question being debated by respiratory physiologists was whether the "true stimulus" to the respiratory center was CO_2 or H^+. But, in fact, Gray really did not answer this question at all, he merely sidestepped it. All equation (4) really says is that if you tell me the values of $[H^+]_a$, P_{aCO_2}, and P_{aO_2}, I will tell you what $\dot{V}_A$ is. It has nothing at all to say about the internal mechanisms through which the respiratory center is ultimately stimulated. Not only that, but as we have previously noted, all of the ventilatory apparatus and the conductive airway intervene between the neural output of the respiratory center and the $\dot{V}_A$ that results. Nevertheless, for the purpose intended, namely, to obtain a useful quantitative description of the chemical control of breathing in men with a normal ventilatory apparatus and gas exchanger, this control law was entirely satisfactory.

To complete this quantitive description of the respiratory chemostat, we have only to close the feedback loops by solving equations (1) through (4) simultaneously. It should be clear in principle that we can do this, and so obtain closed loop equations that will define the dependence of both $\dot{V}_A$ and P_{aCO_2}, $[H^+]_a$, and P_{aO_2} upon particular external or internal disturbances, i.e., CO_2 inhalation (increased P_{iCO_2}), hypoxia (decreased P_{iO_2}), or metabolic disturbances in acid-base balance (altered $[BHCO_3]_{7.4}$). We shall not present these rather complex equations but shall simply summarize their implications in Figures 7-5 through 7-7. The latter show that the actual ventilation in each of the disturbances, CO_2 inhalation (7-5), hypoxia (7-6), and metabolic disturbances of acid-base balance (7-7) is the sum of the partial stimulation and/or inhibition of the three arterial chemical agents, P_{aCO_2}, $[H^+]_a$, and P_{aO_2}.

Metabolic Hyperpnea—Exercise

We have seen how the basic respiratory chemostat gives an illuminating description of the chemical control of breathing and nicely accounts for the behavior observed in CO_2 inhalation, hypoxia, metabolic acidosis, and metabolic alkalosis. All of these might be called compensatory responses in which ventilation changes independently of metabolic rate in order to partially correct for a primary change in one or more of the arterial chemical agents, P_{CO_2},

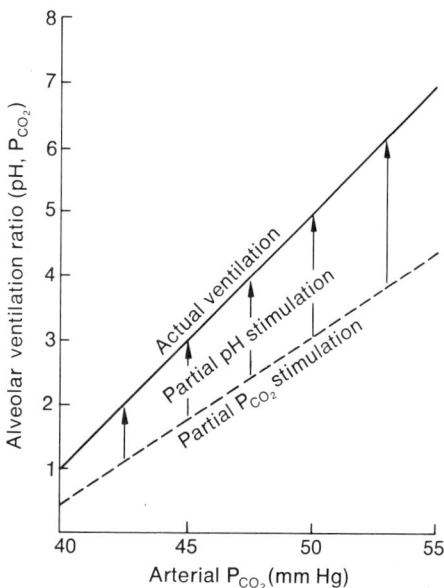

FIGURE 7-5. Closed-loop response of Gray's model to CO_2 inhalation showing additive effects of pH and P_{CO_2}. Alveolar ventilation ratio, VR, is defined as $\dot{V}_A/\dot{V}_{A_0}$. [See equation (4).] (From Gray, John S. *Pulmonary Ventilation and Its Physiological Regulation*, 1950. Courtesy of Charles C Thomas, Publisher, Springfield, Illinois.)

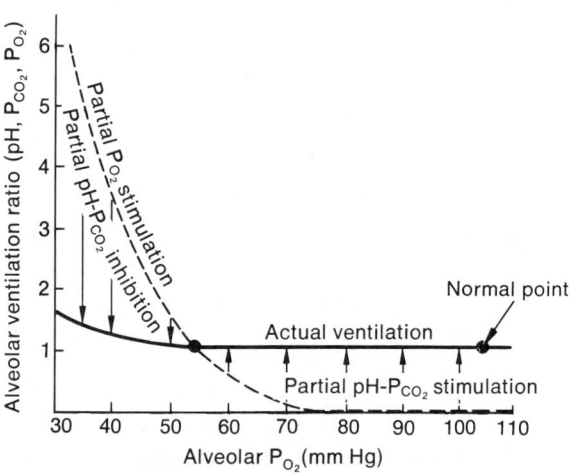

FIGURE 7-6. Response of Gray's model to hypoxia, showing opposition to low P_{O_2} stimulation by pH-P_{CO_2} inhibition. (From Gray, John S. *Pulmonary Ventilation and Its Physiological Regulation*, 1950. Courtesy of Charles C Thomas, Publisher, Springfield, Illinois.)

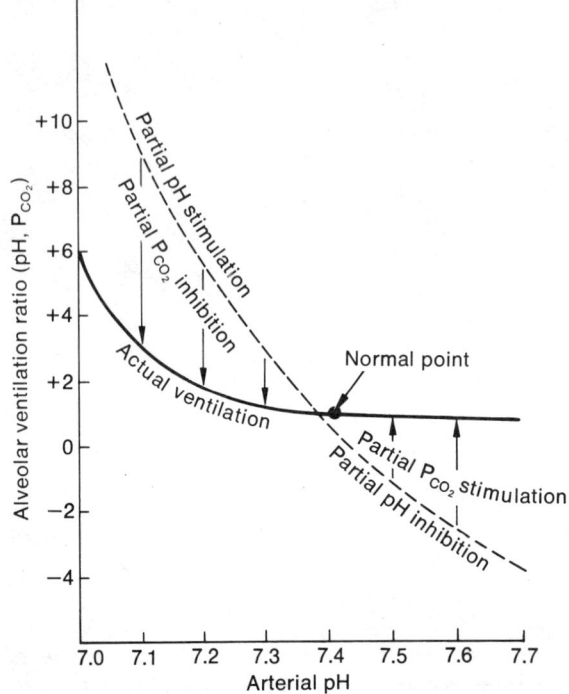

FIGURE 7-7. Response of Gray's model to metabolic disturbances in acid-base balance showing antagonism between pH and P_{CO_2} effects. (From Gray, John S. *Pulmonary Ventilation and Its Physiological Regulation*, 1950. Courtesy of Charles C Thomas, Publisher, Springfield, Illinois.)

P_{O_2}, and [H$^+$]. But what about exercise in which an increase in metabolic rate is the primary disturbance? It should be clear that the basic chemostat shown in Figure 7-3 will respond to exercise by increasing ventilation. Thus a rise in $\dot{V}_{CO_2}$ in equation (1) and in $\dot{V}_{O_2}$ in equation (2) will cause P_{aCO_2} to rise and P_{aO_2} to fall and the rise in P_{aCO_2} will increase [H$^+$]$_a$ through equation (3). All of these changes will stimulate ventilation so that everything appears to be working appropriately to produce the desired ventilatory response. The problem is that if there were no other control mechanism operating, the response would show steady-state errors in P_{aCO_2}, [H$^+$]$_a$, and P_{aO_2}, and this is contrary to the observation that no such errors occur in exercise. So our neat chemical control scheme seems to fail in the most important physiologic situation of all, the hyperpnea of exercise.

We can resort to a simple, *ad hoc* empirical "trick" to resolve this problem. All we have to do is to add another term to our controller law, namely, $k\dot{V}_{CO_2}$. What this implies is that $\dot{V}_{CO_2}$, in addition to providing the material flow of gas into the exchanger already accounted for in equation (1), also provides an "information flow" to the controller that increases $\dot{V}_A$ in proportion to $\dot{V}_{CO_2}$. If $\dot{V}_A$ increases in proportion to $\dot{V}_{CO_2}$ during exercise, then it is clear from equation (1) that P_{aCO_2} will remain constant; i.e., the hyperpnea will be "errorless" as required. The assumption that there is a $k\dot{V}_{CO_2}$ term in the controller law, although it "works" in one sense, is considerably less satisfying physiologically than the other terms in the equation. Even though we may not know the ultimate mechanisms by which the three arterial chemical agents stimulate the respiratory center, we do know that there are reasonably well-defined central and/or peripheral chemoreceptors that do respond to them. But no one knows where to look for the $\dot{V}_{CO_2}$ receptor or how to tell when he has found it! This is really a slight exaggeration, for many studies and suggestions have actually been made to provide a physiologic mechanism for the $k\dot{V}_{CO_2}$ term, ranging from peripheral "ergoreceptors" in exercising muscles to central cortical "radiation" or "arousal" to dynamic P_{aCO_2} oscillations associated with the respiratory cycle. Nevertheless, we must regard this problem as still unresolved at the present time (1978).

This reservation need not dissuade us from adding the practically useful *ad hoc* extension to our block diagram, and we have done this in Figure 7-8. Here we have shown both a material flow and an information flow role for $\dot{V}_{CO_2}$, and we have also explicitly represented the blood buffer component of the plant. In heavy exercise, increased lactic acid production lowers $[BHCO_3]_{7.4}$ to superimpose a metabolic acidosis upon the metabolic hyperpnea of exercise. The modified controller equation corresponding to this diagram is

$$\dot{V}_A = \dot{V}_{A_0}\{0.22[H^+]_a + 0.262 P_{aCO_2} \\ + (105 \times 10^{-0.038 P_{aCO_2}}) + 0.0043 \dot{V}_{CO_2} - 19\} \quad (5)$$

and we can now add a graphic description of the response to exercise to our previous series (Figure 7-9).

Thus the block diagram of Figure 7-8 and the corresponding set of equations (1), (2), (3), and (5) provide a qualitative and quantitative description of the respiratory chemostat applicable to exercise, CO_2 inhalation, hypoxia, and metabolic disturbances in acid-base balance.

CO_2-O_2 Interaction

Although the independence of the P_{aCO_2} and $[H^+]_a$ effects on pulmonary ventilation described by the controller equations (4 and 5) have been generally confirmed (9), it has been shown subsequently

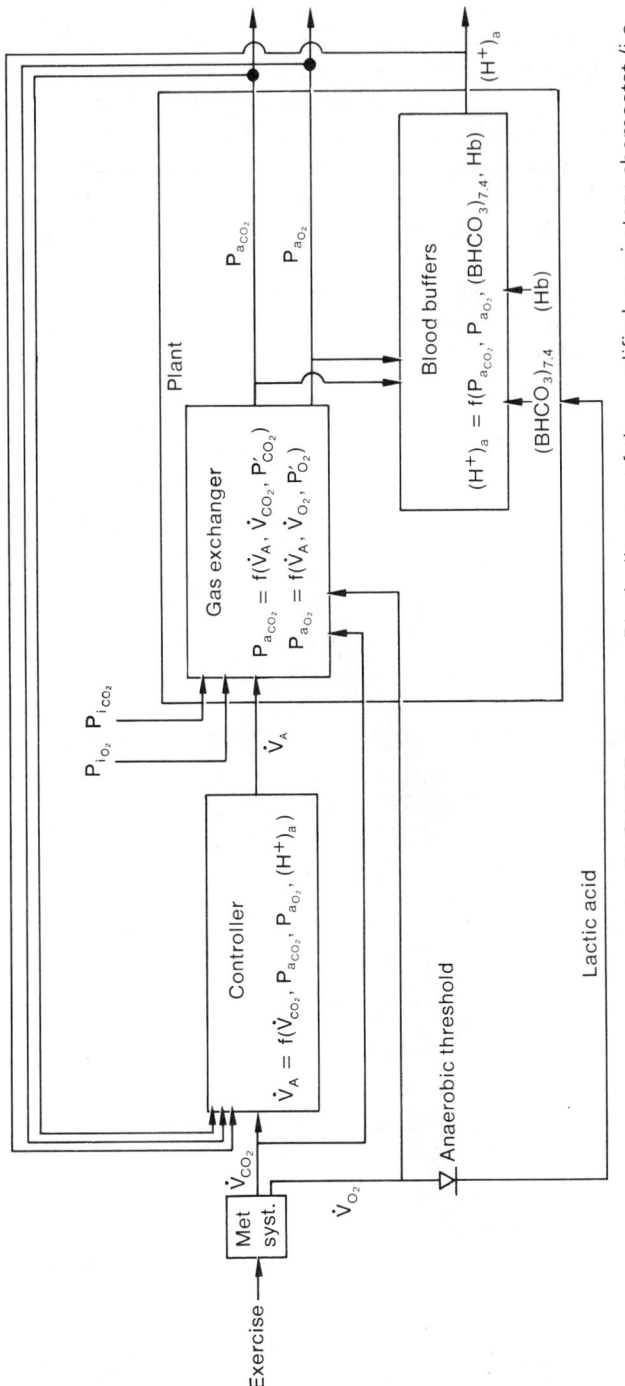

FIGURE 7-8. Block diagram of the modified respiratory chemostat (i.e., the metabolic servomechanism) including a dual role for $\dot{V}_{CO_2}$ (information flow to controller, material flow to gas exchanger).

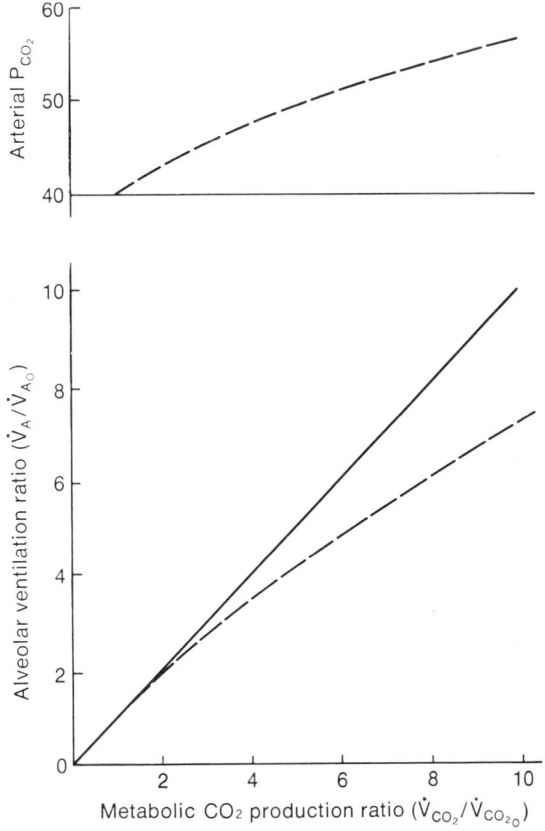

FIGURE 7-9. Response of basic [equation (4), dashed curves] and modified [equation (5), solid curves] respiratory chemostat to moderate exercise.

that there is some interaction between the P_{aCO_2} and P_{aO_2} effects. Thus Nielsen and Smith (47) have examined the ventilatory response to CO_2 inhalation (the *CO_2 response curve*) at three different levels of P_{AO_2} and found that its slope, $\Delta \dot{V}_E/\Delta P_{ACO_2}$, varied with P_{AO_2} (Figure 7-10). Their findings were subsequently confirmed by others (35). Equations (4) and (5) do not describe this observed CO_2-O_2 interaction, and a modified controller equation has been suggested by the Oxford group (Lloyd and Cunningham) to include it:

$$\dot{V} = S(P_{ACO_2} - B) = \left(D + \frac{AD}{P_{AO_2} - C}\right)(P_{ACO_2} - B) \qquad (6)$$

where A, B, C, and D are constants. What this really says is that ventilation is a linear function of P_{ACO_2} with a slope, S, that is itself an

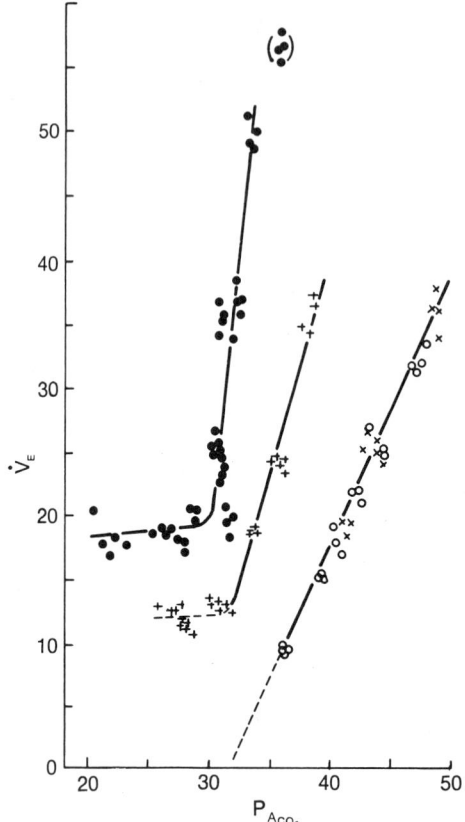

FIGURE 7-10. Ventilation as a function of alveolar P_{CO_2} at three different values of alveolar P_{O_2}: ×, $PA_{O_2} = 169$; ○, $PA_{O_2} = 110$; +, $PA_{O_2} = 47$; ●, $PA_{O_2} = 37$. (From M. Nielson and H. Smith. *Acta Physiol. Scand.* **24**: 293–313, 1952.)

hyperbolic function of $P_{A_{O_2}}$. This is illustrated in Figure 7-11, where the family of CO_2 response curves on the left is frequently referred to as the *Oxford fan*. The major difference between the responses to CO_2 inhalation and hypoxia predicted by equation (6) and Gray's original controller equation (4) occurs in conditions in which hypoxia is combined with hypercapnia. Note also that (6) does not separate out the independent effect of $[H^+]_a$, and so cannot be applied to metabolic disturbances in acid-base balance.

In recent years, interest in the quantitative expression of ventilatory sensitivity to hypercapnia and hypoxia in both normal subjects and patients has increased, and some alternative formulations have appeared (*31, 51, 54*). Since all of these so far are empirical, the choice of which one to use is a matter of personal taste and convenience. However, there have also been some attempts to provide a more

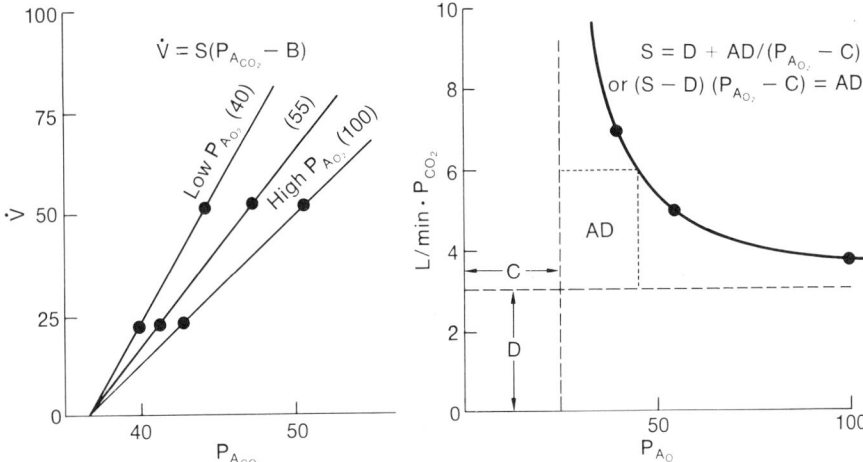

FIGURE 7-11. Idealized representation of CO_2-O_2 interaction. Left: CO_2 response curves represented as a family of straight lines with a common intercept on the abscissa, B, and a slope, S, dependent on P_{AO_2}. Right: Dependence of the slope parameter, S, of the CO_2 response curve on P_{AO_2}. The relationship is hyperbolic. (From *The Regulation of Human Respiration*. Edited by D. J. C. Cunningham and B. B. Lloyd. Oxford: Blackwell Scientific Publications Ltd., 1963, p. 337.)

mechanistic controller equation, and we now briefly examine this question.

Details of Controller Input—Receptor Sites and Stimuli

Although the steady-state, empirical controller equations (4), (5), and (6) are really independent of the actual location of receptor sites or the nature of the ultimate effective stimuli, physiologists have devoted much effort over the years to answering questions of this sort. Of course, any general dynamic description of the control of pulmonary ventilation must depend on knowledge of this kind.

It has been known since the 1930s that low P_{aO_2} stimulates ventilation entirely through the peripheral chemoreceptors in the carotid and aortic bodies (C. J. F. Heymans won the Nobel Prize for this discovery in 1938, a discovery that resolved many years of controversy about the mechanism of hypoxic hyperpnea). On the other hand, it seems equally clear that the steady-state response to CO_2 inhalation is essentially independent of these peripheral receptors, and instead depends on central receptors in the medulla. Just where these receptors are and exactly to what they respond have both been matters of major recent interest and controversy. Thus some have held that they lie on the surface of the medulla and respond primarily to the P_{CO_2} and/or $[H^+]$ of the cerebrospinal fluid (CSF) that bathes them (*44, 45, 46*) whereas others think they lie deeper in the medulla and respond to a local $[H^+]$ that is influenced by the composition of both arterial blood and bulk CSF (*48*). In either case, since CO_2 freely passes the blood-brain barrier, it is easy to see how a rise in P_{aCO_2} could influence these receptors wherever they turn out to be. Although the steady-state response to CO_2 inhalation does not seem to depend at all on the peripheral chemoreceptors, the latter have been shown to respond to rapid dynamic changes in P_{aCO_2}. The significance of this is not clear although it may be involved in the response to exercise (*vide infra*).

The exact mechanism that mediates the ventilatory response to acute and chronic metabolic disturbances in acid-base balance is perhaps not quite so clear. The problem is that H^+, unlike free CO_2, does not readily penetrate the blood-brain barrier and that, at least in acute disturbances, bulk CSF $[H^+]$ either remains constant or changes in a direction opposite to arterial $[H^+]$. The implication is that if there is a "central" $[H^+]$ receptor, it cannot respond only to bulk CSF but either must lie proximal to the blood-brain barrier [cf. Lambertsen (*32*)] or else lie in a special local environment whose $[H^+]$ is strongly influenced by arterial blood composition, presumably through a rapid HCO_3^- flux between blood and a small volume of brain interstitial fluid [cf. Pappenheimer et al. (*48*)]. There is also a peripheral H^+ receptor which, of course, does lie proximal to the blood-brain barrier, i.e., the carotid body. It has been shown that this structure responds to both steady and dynamic changes in $[H^+]_a$, but its contribution to the ventilatory responses to acute metabolic acidosis remains controversial.

Lloyd attempted to express some of these physiologic mechanisms in his *respiratory regulation equation* first proposed in 1966 (*34*). In doing so, he retained some of the general form of his empirical equation (6), but now assumed that all CO_2 effects were mediated by changes in $[H^+]$ at central (medullary) and peripheral arterial (carotid body) receptors. He further assigned all of the CO_2-O_2 interaction expressed in equation (6) to the interaction of $[H^+]_a$ and P_{aO_2} at the carotid body. The equation is

$$\dot{V} = h\left\{\left(\lambda + \log\frac{[H^+]_a}{[H^+]_{a\theta}}\right)\left(\frac{\psi}{P_{aO_2} - \gamma}\right) + \left(\mu + \log\frac{[H^+]_c}{[H^+]_{c\theta}}\right)\right\} \quad (7)$$

where h, λ, γ, ψ, and μ are constants, and $[H^+]_{a\theta}$ and $[H^+]_{c\theta}$ are "threshold" values of arterial and central $[H^+]$, respectively. It is uncertain whether all CO_2-O_2 interaction really is peripheral or whether the equation accounts for metabolic as well as respiratory disturbances in acid-base balance; it is clear that the equation cannot account for the hyperpnea of exercise. We must conclude, therefore, that a satisfactory mechanistic controller equation has yet to be formulated.

We noted on p. 117 that many suggestions have been made for stimuli and receptors to account for the errorless hyperpnea of exercise. Prominent among these are *ergoreceptors* or *metaboloreceptors* in exercising limbs that transmit their information centrally via neural pathways (*29*). Since at the other end of the neural chain it is common knowledge that ventilation can be controlled voluntarily, motor cortical "radiation" or "arousal" spreading to the respiratory center has also been suggested. Finally, dynamic oscillations of P_{aCO_2}, which differ in amplitude in exercise compared to CO_2 inhalation, have also been implicated (*58*). No satisfactory resolution of this problem has yet been achieved.

Finally, we note that there are a whole host of miscellaneous stimuli and conditions that can affect ventilation.

Details of Controller Output—Is $\dot{V}_A$ a Valid Measure?

It has been traditional among respiratory physiologists for many years to assess the "sensitivity" or "gain" of the medullary respiratory controller to particular chemical inputs by measuring their effect on pulmonary ventilation, either total ($\dot{V}_E$) or alveolar ($\dot{V}_A$). The familiar *CO_2 response curve* (Figures 7-10 and 7-11) is an expression of this tradition. But as pointed out on p. 113, there are many unit processes that lie between the motor output of the respiratory center and its ultimate expression as $\dot{V}_E$ or $\dot{V}_A$. Thus the entire ventilatory apparatus, including both its energy source (the respiratory muscles) and its mechanical impedance (resistance, compliance, inertia of lung-thorax and airways), is interposed between motor nerve impulses to the respiratory muscles and $\dot{V}_E$. To get from $\dot{V}_E$ to $\dot{V}_A$, we have to consider the behavior of the conductive airway. Now if we always deal with "normal" people and never impose any external mechanical loads on their ventilatory apparatus, we can learn a good deal about "controller sensitivity" from measurements of $\dot{V}_E$ (or $\dot{V}_A$) even though the *gain coefficients* so obtained (e.g., equations [4] and [5]) really include the characteristics of the ventilatory apparatus (and conductive dead space) in addition to those of the medullary neural controller. Moreover, it is certainly a lot easier to measure pulmonary ventilation than it is to directly measure the neural output of the respiratory center, or to translate the latter, once measured, into an appropriate input to the pulmonary gas exchanger. Thus we hardly need apologize for the traditional method of assessing "controller sensitivity" in normal man.

But if we wish to apply our description of the respiratory chemostat to patients with pulmonary disease, we need to be more careful about what we take as a measure of the controller output if we are to validly distinguish between defects in the controller and defects in the ventilatory apparatus. This can be appreciated even in normal people if we measure their conventional "sensitivity to CO_2" before and after adding a resistive load to the airway. Thus the "reduced sensitivity to CO_2" implied by the results of such a study in Figure 7-12 does not really mean that the load produced a defect in the controller. Considerations such as these have led to a number of suggestions for controller output measurements that, unlike the conventional ventilation, would validly measure controller sensitivity in a wide variety of normal and disease situations. These include the work of breathing (not particularly easy to measure in man), which is shown in Figure 7-12; some sort of integrated phrenic neurograms or diaphragmatic or intercostal electromyograms (*11, 39*) (not particularly easy either); and, most recently, the *occlusion pressure* developed 100 msec from the start of inspiration against a closed airway, P_{100} (*55*). It remains to be seen how useful any of these will turn out to be, but the need for some such measurement is clear enough.

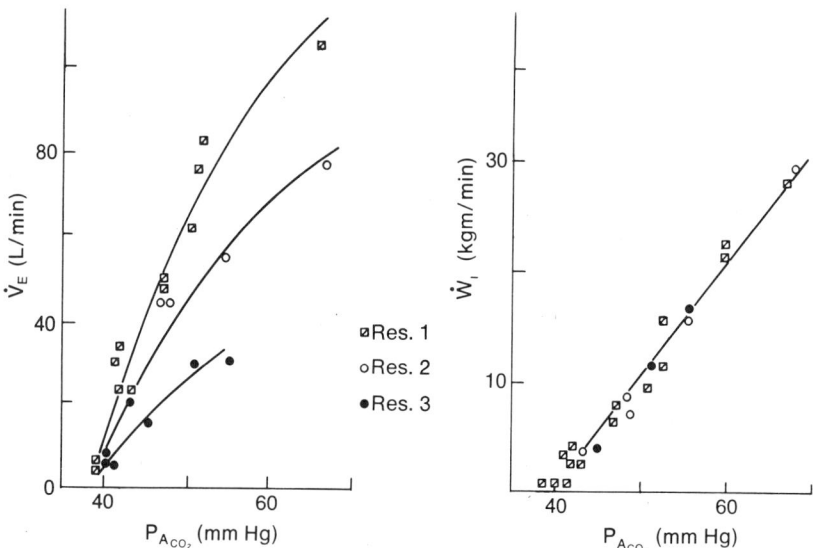

FIGURE 7-12. Effect of added airway resistance on conventional CO_2 response curve (left) and on the same curves transformed from ventilation to inspiratory work rate (right). [Modified from J. Milic-Emili and J. M. Tyler. *J. Appl. Physiol.* **18**(3): 497–504, 1963.]

Complications in the Plant—The "Expanded Chemostat"

Again, if our description of the respiratory chemostat is to be useful in understanding the control of ventilation in patients with pulmonary disease, we need to reexamine some of the assumptions that Gray originally made to simplify his description of the normal gas exchanger. Thus we know from Chapter 4 that $P_{a_{O_2}}$ does not equal $P_{A_{O_2}}$ or $P_{e_{O_2}}$ even in normal people, and that in pulmonary disease, $\dot{V}_e$ may not equal $\dot{V}_A$ nor $P_{a_{CO_2}}$ equal $P_{A_{CO_2}}$. It is clear that what we really need to do is to incorporate the detailed descriptions of both the ventilatory apparatus (Chapter 3) and the pulmonary gas exchanger (Chapter 4) into an expanded description of the respiratory chemostat that will make it generally applicable to both normal people and patients with pulmonary disease.

This is a formidable task, and for the purposes of this book we shall content ourselves with the simplified diagramatic representation shown in Figure 7-13. It is clear that to adequately understand and characterize the normal as well as the abnormal system, we must describe the quantitative characteristics of each unit process in Figure 7-13 as best we can. We shall rarely be able to do it completely, but it is nevertheless useful to know what we are aiming for.

The Respiratory Cycle

In the present chapter we have carefully described the control of pulmonary ventilation without once mentioning its most obvious feature, i.e., that ventilation is a periodic process. We all know, of course, that we do not ventilate our lungs via a unidirectional, continuous flow of air but rather by an alternating inflation and deflation of the lung-thorax "bellows." Thus pulmonary ventilation is a cyclic process in which the average minute ventilation is the product of respiratory frequency and tidal volume. Moreover, it is clear that a given ventilation ordered by our metabolic servosystem could be achieved by a variety of such frequency-tidal volume combinations so that it is natural to ask what factors determine the particular choice the system makes. It is perhaps a historical accident in respiratory physiology that those primarily interested in the "chemical control of breathing" generally ignore the respiratory cycle and talk only about "pulmonary ventilation," whereas those primarily interested in the "neural control of breathing" generally ignore its chemistry and concentrate on the neural mechanisms responsible for its periodicity. Fortunately, the organism has been able to bring these two aspects together although

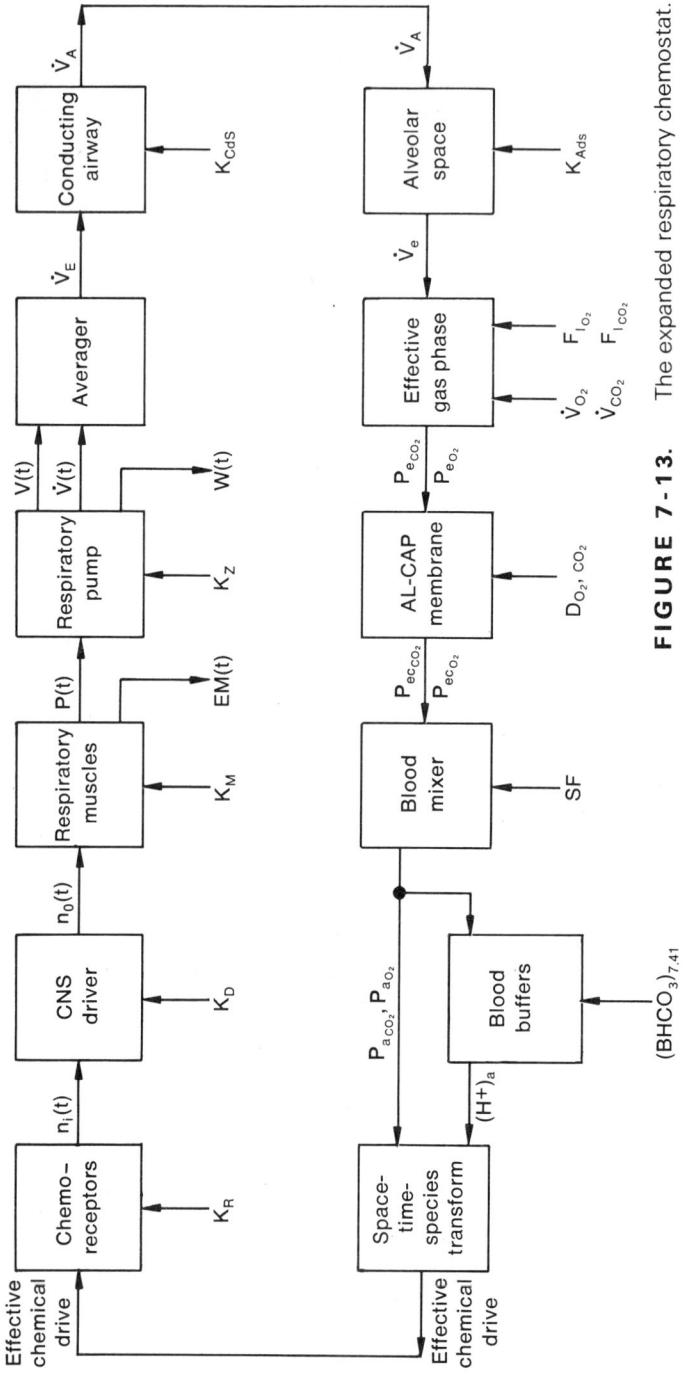

FIGURE 7-13. The expanded respiratory chemostat.

respiratory physiologists in general have not. However, very recently there are signs that this essential integration may be beginning.

Let us begin our discussion by examining the basic neural components that are responsible for the origin and modulation of the respiratory cycle, and then examine some models that start to bring "chemical" and "neural" control together into a single comprehensive scheme.

BASIC NEURAL CIRCUIT COMPONENTS

INVOLUNTARY SYSTEM. It has long been known that neural centers essential for automatic, involuntary respiration are present in the medulla. Recent studies have located them in the vicinity of the nucleus of the solitary tract (dorsal respiratory group), and the nuclei ambiguus and retroambigualis (ventral respiratory group) (Figure 7-14). Most axons from these medullary centers cross in the medulla

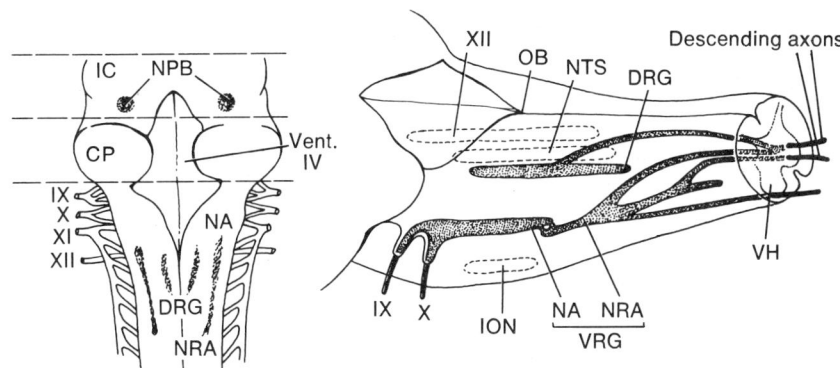

FIGURE 7-14. Dorsal (A) and dorso-lateral (B) views of cat brain stem to show the dorsal (DRG) and ventral (VRG) respiratory groups and their projections. NPB, nucleus parabrachialis; IC, inferior colliculus; CP, cerebellar peduncle; NA, nucleus ambiguus; NRA, nucleus retroambigualis, OB, OBEX; NTS, nucleus tractus solitarius; ion, inf. olivary nuc.; VH, ventral horn. (Modified from R. A. Mitchell and A. J. Berger. *Ann. Rev. Respir. Dis.* **111**: 206–224, 1975.)

and descend in the ventral and lateral columns to spinal segmental levels (Figure 7-15). Although denied by earlier work, it has now been established that the medulla is not only necessary but is also sufficient for involuntary breathing. This means that the medullary complex contains a self-oscillator (or central pattern generator, CPG) that will convert a steady chemical drive into a periodic motor discharge even when isolated from all other neural inputs. Although the detailed mechanisms responsible for this property remain unknown, the

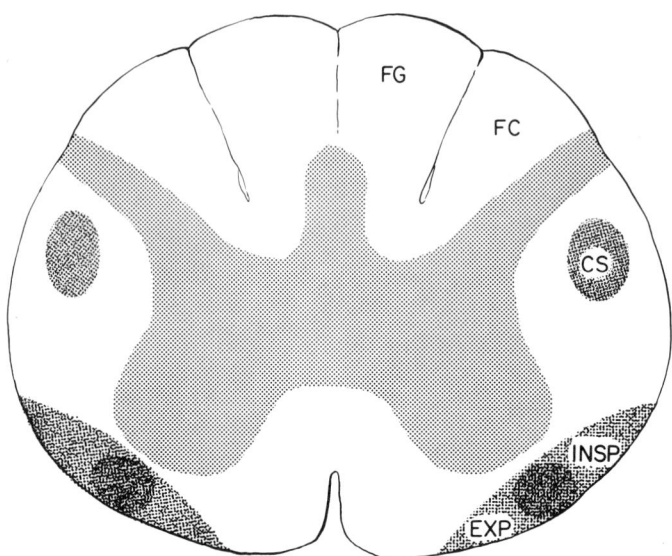

FIGURE 7-15. Location of the descending respiratory pathways in the cervical cord of cat. Voluntary control in corticospinal tracts (CS). Involuntary pathways both rhythmic and nonrhythmic lie in the ventral and lateral columns indicated by crosshatch regions. The descending expiratory axons (EXP) tend to be medial to inspiratory axons (INS). Other abbreviations: FG, funiculus gracilis; FC, funiculus cuneatus. (From R. A. Mitchell and A. J. Berger. *Ann. Rev. Respir. Dis.* **111**: 206–224, 1975.)

medulla acts as if it contained a switch that can interrupt the respiratory drive or direct it alternately to generators of inspiratory (central inspiratory activity, CIA or CIE) or expiratory (CEA) activity. Although still speculative, the CIA most probably lies in the nucleus of the solitary tract as does the inspiratory off switch. Much less is known about the CEA generator, but it is probably associated with the ventral respiratory group.

In the intact animal, the activity of this basic medullary oscillator is modulated by neural inputs from both higher brain centers (pneumotaxic center in the nucleus parabrachialis, NPB, in the pons; apneustic center in the nucleus reticularis gigantocellularis and rostral nucleus reticularis ventralis of the upper medulla) and from peripheral pulmonary stretch receptors via the vagi as we shall describe in a moment.

VOLUNTARY SYSTEM. Impulses mediating voluntary control of breathing arise from the motor and premotor cortex and descend in the corticospinal tracts (Figure 7-15). Thus voluntary and involuntary breathing are mediated by two different systems that are anatomically separate at all sites in the corticospinal axis down to the segmental level in the spinal cord where they project to spinal respiratory motoneurons.

The basic neural circuitry comprising the voluntary and involuntary systems is summarized in the block diagram of Figure 7-16. Starting with the normal respiratory cycle in the intact animal, we can examine the effects of selective interruption of the modulating neural inputs. The nature and influence of vagal feedback from the lungs was first described by Hering and Breuer in 1868. Stretch receptors in the lung increase their discharge rate as lung volume increases during inspiration, and this information, transmitted to the medulla via the vagi, terminates inspiration and initiates expiration. If this volume feedback signal is interrupted by bilateral vagotomy, tidal volume increases markedly and frequency decreases with little change in total ventilation. In terms of the medullary switching mechanism shown in Figure 7-16, the volume feedback signal throws the switch from its inspiratory position at a smaller tidal volume (and hence sooner) than would otherwise occur. The pulmonary stretch receptors responsible for this volume feedback have been shown to lie in the smooth muscle of the airways.

As previously noted, the respiratory cycle is also modulated by influences from higher centers as revealed by the effects of brain stem transections. A midpontine transection that interrupts only the pneumotaxic center input to the medulla produces slow, deep breathing much like that seen after vagotomy. We interpret this to mean that the pneumotaxic center input normally facilitates the ability of vagal feedback to throw the medullary switch and terminate inspiration as indicated by the + sign in Figure 7-16. If this midpontine section is combined with bilateral vagotomy, so-called "apneustic" breathing results. This is characterized by extremely prolonged end inspiratory pauses; the chest may remain inflated for several minutes before one or two quick expirations break through to be followed by another prolonged apneusis. If 100% O_2 is given to permit survival of the animal, the apneustic breaths gradually become shorter, but end-inspiratory pauses persist. It is as if the medullary oscillator finds it very difficult to throw the unfacilitated switch without vagal feedback and the switch "sticks" in its preferred inspiratory position. However, more recent work suggests that the apneustic center does not affect the medullary oscillator directly at all but instead operates through long reticulospinal fibers that excite inspiratory and inhibit expiratory motor neurons at the spinal cord level. We have included both possibilities in the dashed, question-marked connections from the apneustic center in Figure 7-16. The negative sign at the switch input means that it normally inhibits throwing the switch from inspiration to expiration.

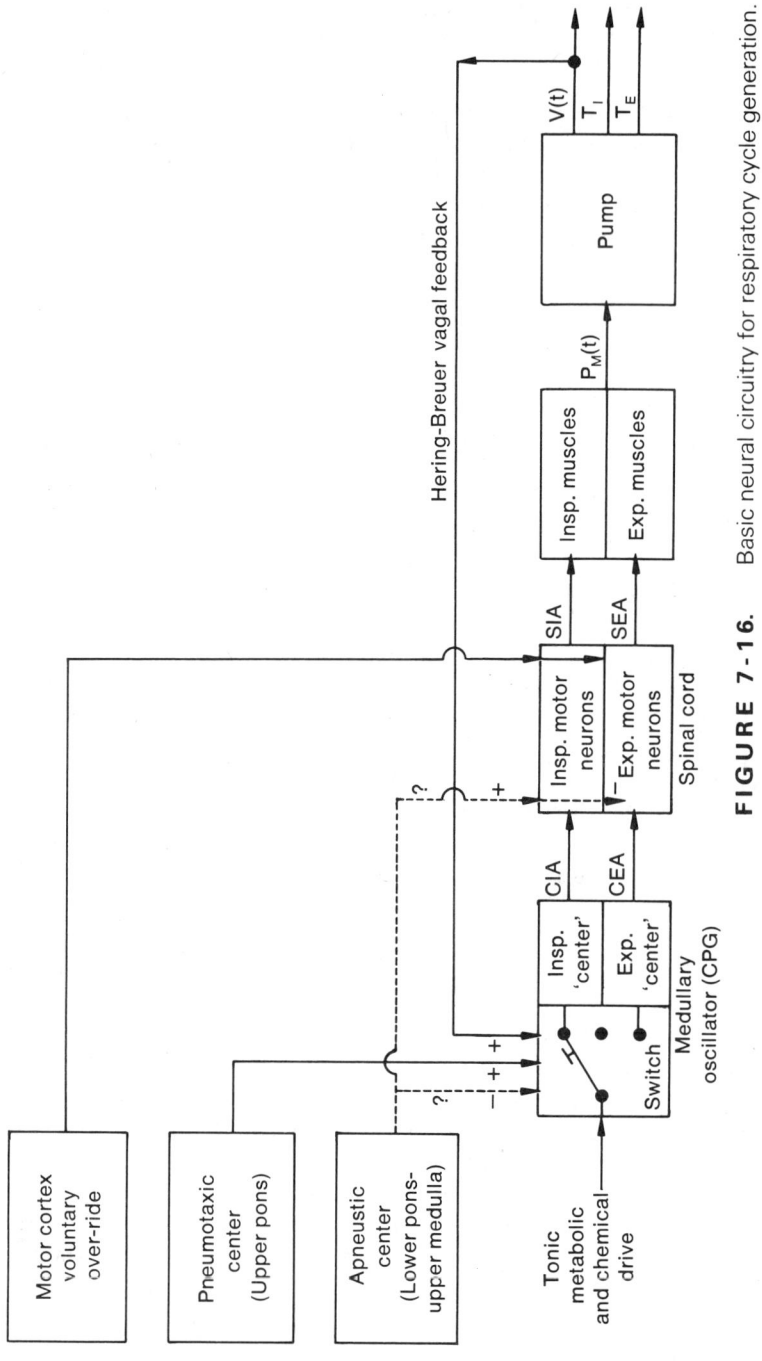

FIGURE 7-16. Basic neural circuitry for respiratory cycle generation.

If we now make a lower transection at the medullary-pontine junction, depending on the exact level of the transection, apneustic breathing is replaced either by an essentially normal pattern or by "ataxic" breathing. The latter is a somewhat irregular cyclic pattern characterized by quick inspiratory gasps followed by end expiratory pauses. Presumably, elimination of apneustic inhibition of expiration, either at the switch or spinal cord levels, restores the basic medullary rhythm. The apneustic breathing pattern is rarely, if ever, seen clinically. However, ataxic breathing does appear in deep respiratory depression (narcotics, anesthesia; e.g., it is commonly seen in dogs under nembutal), or in damage to the brain stem by trauma or ischemia, and is a common form of terminal breathing.

It is, of course, common knowledge that the breathing pattern and ventilation can be altered by voluntary effort, and we have shown such a "voluntary override" pathway from the motor cortex to the spinal motoneurons in Figure 7-16. As previously noted, the voluntary control path is completely separate from the involuntary one so that the two systems may be independently damaged by appropriately placed CNS lesions either experimentally or in disease.

QUANTITATIVE FEATURES OF CYCLE BEHAVIOR

In recent years there has been renewed interest in the regulation of the rate and depth of breathing and the role of the Hering-Breuer reflex in man. We shall consider two aspects of these developments.

THE "HEY PLOT." When ventilation increases in normal man in response to either exercise, CO_2 inhalation, or hypoxia, both frequency and tidal volume increase. If ventilation is plotted as a function of tidal volume (Figure 7-17), the relationship is identical for all three forcings, being linear up to a tidal volume of about 2.5 liters (or 50% of vital capacity) after which it turns almost vertically upward; i.e., further increase in ventilation is accomplished by increasing frequency only with V_T remaining constant. Figure 7-17 is known as the "Hey plot," having been introduced by Hey, Lloyd, Cunningham, Jukes, and Bolton in 1966 and widely adopted since as a convenient way to summarize the behavior of cycle pattern as $\dot{V}$ increases. It is of interest that the Hey plot is not generally influenced by the nature of respiratory stimulus although increased body temperature is an exception to this. Also, in diseases of the lung such as pneumonia, frequency may increase greatly while tidal volume falls (*vide infra*).

THE CLARK-VON EULER MODEL. In 1972, Clark and von Euler proposed the model shown in Figure 7-18 to explain the way in which

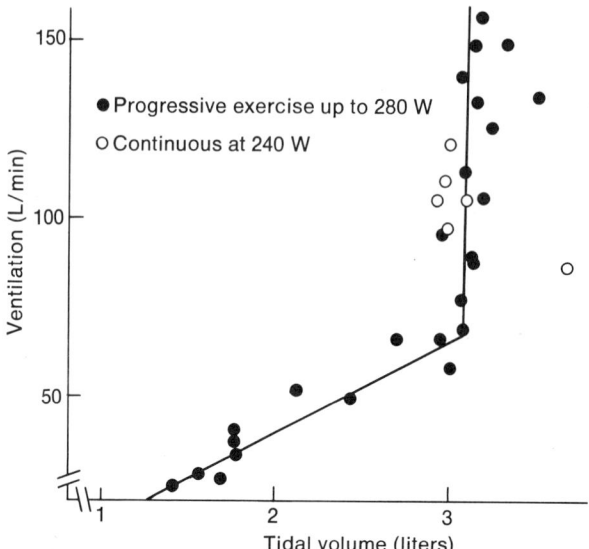

FIGURE 7-17. The Hey plot. Relationship of ventilation to tidal volume in a normal subject (R. S.) during exercise on a cycle ergometer. W = watts. (From J. E. Cotes, G. R. Johnson, and A. McDonald. In: *Breathing: Hering-Breuer Centenary Symposium.* Edited by Ruth Porter. London: J. & A. Churchill, 1970.)

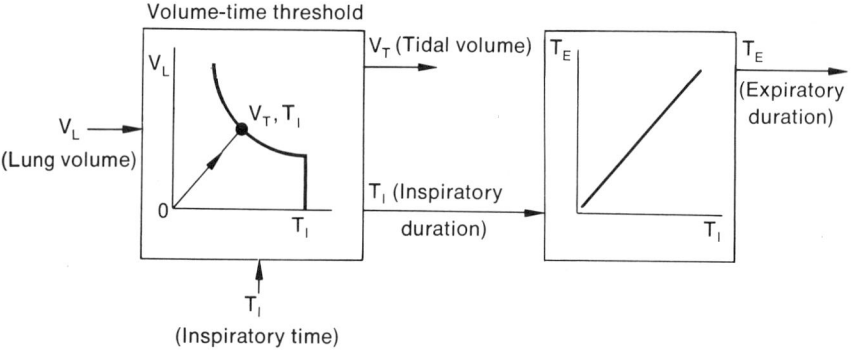

FIGURE 7-18. Clark-von Euler model of cycle control.

vagal volume feedback determines tidal volume, V_T, inspiratory duration, T_I, and expiratory duration, T_E. Lung volume, V_L, is assumed to increase during inspiration at a rate fixed by chemical drive. Inspiration terminates and expiration begins (i.e., the inspiratory off-switch is thrown) when the linearly rising V_L intersects a *volume-time threshold curve* whose shape is determined by both vagal feedback and the properties of the medullary oscillator. Three ranges of operation are recognized. In range 1, which includes low tidal volumes, vagal feedback is ineffective and the curve is vertical, i.e., any increase in $\dot{V}$ is accomplished by increases in V_T alone with f remaining constant at a relatively low value representing the natural frequency of the respiratory oscillator. In range 2 (the *Hering-Breuer range*), the curve is hyperbolic and expresses the notion that the volume threshold for termination of inspiration by vagal feedback decreases with time from the onset of inspiration. If the vagi are cut, this hyperbolic range 2 is replaced by an extension of the vertical range 1 to high tidal volumes. This description is compatible with recent findings that the Hering-Breuer reflex is apparently inactive during eupneic breaking in awake man, since vagal block by local anesthesia does not alter the respiratory cycle. Apparently, eupneic awake man operates in range 1. However, if ventilation is increased by CO_2 inhalation, awake man operates in range 2, and now vagal block will produce the slowing and deepening of breathing typically seen following vagotomy in anesthetized animals. A range 3 has been described at high tidal volumes although its exact shape is still uncertain. To explain the vertical portion of the Hey plot (Figure 7-17), one would expect range 3 to be horizontal and extend to low values of T_I. However, this is not the shape originally described by Clark and von Euler, and this point remains to be resolved.

More recent studies by von Euler and his associates have extended this model and elucidated some of its underlying neurophysiology. Central inspiratory excitation (CIE) probably originates in the inspiratory spinal (IS) cells of the ventrolateral nucleus of the solitary tract. Left to itself, this CIE rises as a ramp function superimposed on an initial step that terminates abruptly when it reaches a fixed threshold. Sensory vagal input can do only one thing, i.e., it can terminate the CIE prematurely. The off-trigger signal is thought to arise in the inspiratory vagal (IV) cells of the nucleus of the solitary tract whenever the sum of CIE and vagal volume feedback reaches a fixed threshold. Since CIE rises as a ramp function during inspiration, the vagal feedback required to reach the trigger threshold falls linearly with time (cf. the volume-time threshold curve in Figure 7-18). This concept of the basic operation of the inspiratory off-switch is shown diagrammatically in Figure 7-19, and some postulated neurophysiologic circuits are shown in Figure 7-20.

To account for the initial steplike rise in CIE preceding the ramp, it has recently been postulated that the CIE is separable into two components, a tonic component represented by the initial step function whose magnitude depends on tonic drives such as CO_2, and a superimposed ramp function whose slope is more or less independent of such drives. To account for the facts that CO_2 breathing increases

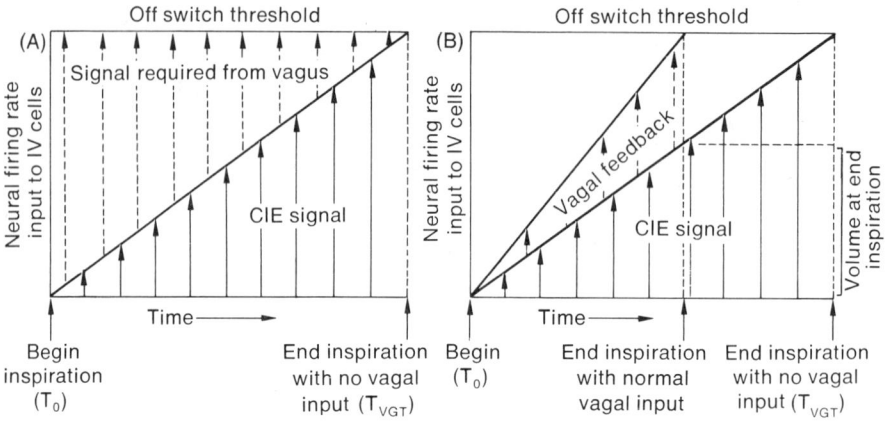

FIGURE 7-19. Operation of the inspiratory off switch. The diagram shows the inputs to the IV cells. The threshold at which the IV cells generate the off switch is shown as constant during a breath. (A) The CIE signal increases continuously. It alone will eventually cause the IV cells to reach off-switch threshold. Inspiration then terminates at the CPG duration, as seen after vagotomy, T_{VGT}. At any time earlier than this a sufficient lung inflation signal can sum with the CIE and cause the IV cells to reach off threshold early. The volume feedback required to reach the off-switch threshold decreases with time from beginning of inspiration. (B) With the vagi intact the lung volume feedback signal sums with the CIE and the off threshold is reached earlier. The volume of the lungs at any time is roughly proportional to the CIE signal. The lung volume attained at inspiratory cut off with normal vagal input is marked at the right of the graph. The volume attained without vagal feedback would be proportional to the full length of the vertical axis. (From R. J. Wyman. *Ann. Rev. Physiol.* **39**: 417–448, 1977. Reproduced, with permission, from the *Annual Review of Physiology,* Volume 39. Copyright © 1977 by Annual Reviews Inc. All rights reserved.)

both the rate and depth of breathing in the intact animal but only the depth after vagotomy, it has been proposed that increased CO_2 not only increases the magnitude of the CIE step but also inhibits the IV cells by an equal amount, so that, in effect, the off-switch threshold is raised. This concept is shown diagrammatically in Figure 7-21. Some sort of similar assumption that makes the vagal feedback required to trigger the off-switch constant and independent of T_I when $V_T \geq 2.5$ liters in man would seem to be necessary to account for the Hey plot.

This recent work is a long step forward in the eventual integration of our understanding of neural and chemical control. However, much remains to be learned. Thus, although we have some understanding of how CIE is turned off, we really do not know how it is turned on or what determines its form. We do not know what determines T_E. Although Clark and von Euler postulated that it was proportional to T_I (see Figure 7-18), this is contrary to recent experimental findings. We

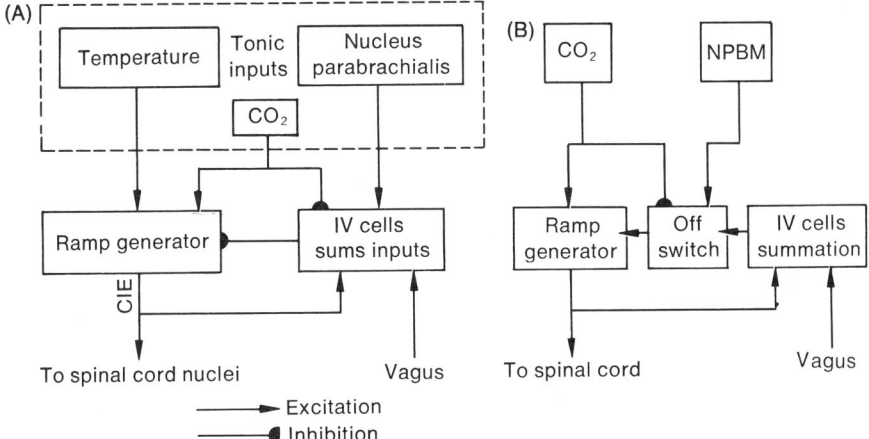

FIGURE 7-20. (A) Simplest network to explain Hering-Breuer reflex. The CIE ramp activity sums in the IV cells with impulses from the slowly adapting lung stretch receptors traveling in the vagus nerve. At a certain value of the sum, the IV cells send an inspiration terminating off trigger to the ramp generator. Tonic inputs are described in the text; they contribute a tonic drive or inhibition to the ramp generator and/or the IV cells. (B) Alternative model for the off switch. This model interposes a separate group of off-switch neurons between the IV cells and the ramp generator. In this model, CO_2 and NPBM input play on the off-switch cells instead of the IV cells. Similar to a model of Bradley et al. (18). (From R. J. Wyman. *Ann. Rev. Physiol.* **39**: 417–448, 1977. Reproduced, with permission, from the *Annual Review of Physiology*, Volume 39. Copyright ©1977 by Annual Reviews Inc. All rights reserved.)

do not know whether CIE is generated by pacemaker cells similar to those found in invertebrates or whether this self-oscillation depends on a network of neurons with appropriate interconnections. We do know that a reciprocally inhibiting network involving inspiratory and expiratory cell populations that has been postulated in the past is probably not involved. The required interconnections have not been found except at the spinal cord level. We know very little about the origin of active expiration or how it is terminated.

Thus we look forward to the clarification of these and other questions in the future.

Other Receptors in the Lung

Beside the stretch receptors that provide volume feedback for the Hering-Breuer reflex, a number of other pulmonary receptors have been described. These include *irritant receptors* and *J receptors* (or *juxta pulmonary capillary receptors*). The former are thought to lie in

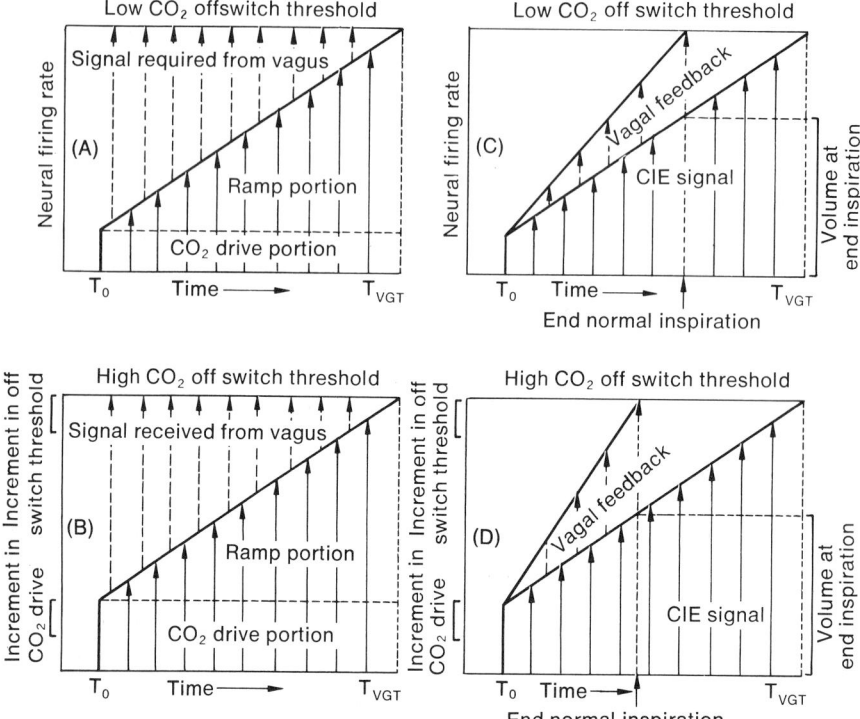

FIGURE 7-21. Effect of CO_2 in the model of Figure 7.20B. (A) CO_2 is considered to add a tonic baseline component to the CIE activity. The total CIE, then, is the firing rate, indicated by solid arrows as the sum of the CO_2 drive portion and the ramp generator portion. The IV cells receive this CIE as input. (B) At higher CO_2 levels the baseline CO_2 activity is increased. The ramp component is unchanged by CO_2. In addition, the off-switch cells are inhibited tonically by CO_2, thus at high CO_2 the off-switch threshold is higher. However, since the CIE and the off-switch threshold are raised equally, the difference between the two is unchanged and is independent of CO_2 level. Thus, as seen in (A) and (B) the signal required from the vagus to terminate inspiration (volume-threshold curve) is independent of CO_2 level. Duration of inspiration after vagotomy (T_{VGT}) is also independent of CO_2 level. (C) and (D) The vagal feedback at low and high CO_2 is shown in these diagrams. Since the lungs expand more rapidly at high CO_2 (D), the vagal feedback also increases more rapidly than at low CO_2 (C). The CIE and vagal feedback sum to reach the off threshold earlier at high CO_2 (D) than at low CO_2 (C). Thus, with vagal feedback intact, CO_2 produces faster and deeper breaths. (From R. J. Wyman. *Ann. Rev. Physiol.* **39**: 417–448, 1977. Reproduced, with permission, from the *Annual Review of Physiology*, Volume 39, Copyright © 1977 by Annual Reviews Inc. All rights reserved.)

the epithelium of the airways from the trachea to the respiratory bronchioles and produce reflex hyperpnea and bronchoconstriction in response to inhalation of chemical or mechanical irritants. They are also stimulated by deflation of the lungs and may be responsible for the spontaneous deep breaths seen in most mammals. The J receptors are thought to lie in the alveolar walls adjacent to the pulmonary capillaries and are stimulated by pulmonary congestion, edema, microembolism, pneumonia, and inhalation of irritants. Typically, they produce reflex apnea followed by rapid shallow breathing as well as hypotension and bradycardia. Thus both irritant and J receptors respond primarily to nociceptive agents and probably do not play any significant role in the normal vagal modulation of the respiratory cycle. However, the vagal reflexes originating from them are very important in interpreting the altered patterns that are seen in disease. Thus the J receptors are probably responsible for the tachypnea seen in pneumonia and in pulmonary congestion and microembolism. Like the stretch receptors, both irritant and J receptor afferents travel in the vagi.

Periodic Breathing

Under certain conditions, ventilation may gradually wax and wane in an alternating pattern called periodic or Cheyne-Stokes breathing. This phenomenon represents an instability in the chemical control of ventilation rather than in the cycle control system. There are only two factors that, by themselves, can produce such instability:

1. Increased controller sensitivity to CO_2, which may or may not result from hypoxia.
2. Increased blood circulation time, which increases the transport delay between the lungs and chemoreceptors.

Bouts of periodic breathing may be set off by the hypoxia of altitude or by a variety of temporary disturbances of breathing. Persistent periodic breathing (i.e., Cheyne-Stokes) may occur in cardiac or pulmonary disease and, when it does, it indicates a poor prognosis.

References

1. Band, D. M., I. R. Cameron, and S. J. G. Semple. The effect on respiration of abrupt changes in carotid artery pH and P_{CO_2} in the cat. *J. Physiol. (Lond.)* **211**: 479–494, 1970.

2. Biscoe, T. J. Carotid body: Structure and function. *Physiol. Rev.* **51**: 427–495, 1971.
3. Bradley, G. W., C. von Euler, I. Marttila, and B. Roos. A model of the control and reflex inhibition of inspiration in the cat. *Biol. Cybernetics* **19**: 106–116, 1975.
4. Breuer, J. Self-steering of respiration through the nervus vagus. Translated by E. Ullman. In: *Breathing: Hering-Breuer Centenary Symposium*. Edited by R. Porter. London: J. & A. Churchill, 1970, pp. 365–394.
5. Clark, F. J., and C. von Euler. On the regulation of depth and rate of breathing. *J. Physiol.* **222**: 267–295, 1972.
6. Cotes, J. E., G. R. Johnson, and A. McDonald. Breathing frequency and tidal volume: Relationship to breathlessness. In: *Breathing: Hering-Breuer Centenary Symposium*. Edited by R. Porter. London: J. & A. Churchill, 1970, pp. 297–314.
7. Cunningham, D. J. C. Integrative aspects of the regulation of breathing: A personal view. In: *MTP International Review of Science, Physiology, Series 1, Vol. 2, Respiratory Physiology*. Edited by J. G. Widdicombe. London: Thornton Butterworth Ltd., 1974, pp. 303–369.
8. Cunningham, D. J. C. The control system regulating breathing in man. *Q. Rev. Biophys.* **6**: 433–483, 1974.
9. Domizi, D. B., J. F. Perkins, Jr., and J. S. Byrne. Ventilatory responses to fixed acid evaluated by "iso-P_{CO_2}" technique. *J. Appl. Physiol.* **14**: 557–561, 1959.
10. Dutton, R. E., and S. Permutt. Ventilatory response to transient changes in carbon dioxide. In: *Arterial Chemoreceptors*. Edited by R. W. Torrance. Oxford: Blackwell Scientific Publications Ltd., 1968.
11. Eldridge, F. L. The relationship between phrenic nerve activity and ventilation. *Am. J. Physiol.* **221**: 535–543, 1971.
12. Fencl, V., T. B. Miller, and J. R. Pappenheimer. Studies on the respiratory response to disturbances of acid-base balance, with deductions concerning the ionic composition of cerebral interstitial fluid. *Am. J. Physiol.* **210**: 459–472, 1966.
13. Gelfand, R., and C. J. Lambertsen. Dynamic respiratory response to abrupt change of inspired CO_2 at normal and high P_{O_2}. *J. Appl. Physiol.* **35**: 903–913, 1973.
14. Gesell, R. The chemical regulation of respiration. *Physiol. Rev.* **6**: 551, 1925.
15. Gray, J. S. The multiple factor theory of the control of respiratory ventilation. *Science* **103**: 739–744, 1946.
16. Gray, J. S. *Pulmonary Ventilation and Its Physiological Regulation*. Springfield, Ill.: Charles C Thomas, Publisher, 1950.
17. Grodins, F. S. Analysis of factors concerned in regulation of breathing in exercise. *Physiol. Rev.* **30**: 220–239, 1950.
18. Grodins, F. S. *Control Theory and Biological Systems*. New York: Columbia University Press, 1963.
19. Grodins, F. S. Regulation of pulmonary ventilation. *Physiologist* **7**: 319–333, 1964.
20. Grodins, F. S. Questions and answers about the control of breathing. In:

Regulation and Control in Physiological Systems. Edited by A. S. Iberall and A. C. Guyton. Pittsburgh: Instrument Society of America, 1973.

21. Grodins, F. S., J. Buell, and A. J. Bart. Mathematical analysis and digital simulation of the respiratory control system, *J. Appl. Physiol.* **22**: 260–276, 1967.
22. Grodins, F. S., J. S. Gray, K. R. Schroeder, A. L. Norins, and R. W. Jones. Respiratory responses to CO_2 inhalation: A theoretical study of a nonlinear biological regulator. *J. Appl. Physiol.* **7**: 283–308, 1954.
23. Grodins, F. S., and G. James. Mathematical models of respiratory regulation. *Ann. N.Y. Acad. Sci.* **109**: 852–868, 1963.
24. Grodins, F. S., and S. M. Yamashiro. Control of ventilation. In: *Lung Biology in Health and Disease* (Executive Editor, Claude Lenfant), Vol. 3, *Bioengineering Aspects of the Lung.* Edited by J. B. West. New York: Marcel Dekker, Inc., 1977, p. 515.
25. Haldane, J. S., and J. G. Priestley. The regulation of the lung ventilation. *J. Physiol. (Lond.)* **32**: 225–266, 1905.
26. Hering, E. Self-steering of respiration through the nervus vagus. Translated by E. Ullmann. In: *Breathing: Hering-Breuer Centenary Symposium.* Edited by R. Porter. London: J. & A. Churchill, 1970, pp. 365–394.
27. Hey, E. N., B. B. Lloyd, D. J. C. Cunningham, M. G. M. Jukes, and D. P. G. Bolton. Effects of various respiratory stimuli on the depth and frequency of breathing in man. *Respir. Physiol.* **1**: 193–205, 1966.
28. Hornbein, T. F., and S. C. Sorensen. The chemical regulation of ventilation. In: *Physiology and Biophysics*, 20th ed., Vol. 2. Edited by T. C. Ruch and H. D. Patton. Philadelphia: W. B. Saunders Company, 1974.
29. Kao, F. F. An experimental study of the pathways involved in exercise hyperpnea employing cross-circulation techniques. In: *The Regulation of Human Respiration.* Edited by D. J. C. Cunningham and B. B. Lloyd. Oxford: Blackwell Scientific Publications Ltd., 1963.
30. Kellog, R. H. Central chemical regulation of respiration. In: *Handbook of Physiology*, Section 3, *Respiration*, Vol. 1. Edited by W. O. Fenn and H. Rahn. Washington: American Physiology Society, 1964, p. 507.
31. Kronenberg, R., F. N. Hamilton, R. Gabel, R. Hickey, D. J. C. Read, and J. Seveninghaus. Comparison of three methods for quantitating respiratory responses to hypoxia in man. *Respir. Physiol.* **16**: 109–125, 1972.
32. Lambertsen, C. J. Respiration. In: *Medical Physiology*, 13th ed. Edited by V. B. Mountcastle. St. Louis, Mo.: The C. V. Mosby Company, 1974, p. 58.
33. Leusen, I. Regulation of cerebrospinal fluid composition with reference to breathing. *Physiol. Rev.* **52**: 1–56, 1972.
34. Lloyd, B. B. The interactions between hypoxia and other ventilatory stimuli. In: *International Symposium on the Cardiovascular and Respiratory Effects of Hypoxia.* Edited by J. D. Hatcher and D. B. Jennings. Basel, Switzerland: Karger, 1966.
35. Lloyd, B. B., and D. J. C. Cunningham. A quantitative approach to the regulation of human respiration. In: *The Regulation of Human Respiration.* Edited by D. J. C. Cunningham and B. B. Lloyd. Oxford: Blackwell Scientific Publications Ltd., 1963.

36. Loeschcke, H. H. The respiratory control system: Analysis of steady state solutions for metabolic and respiratory acidosis-alkalosis and increased metabolism. *Pflugers Arch.* 341: 23–42, 1973.
37. Loeschcke, H. H., and K. H. Gertz. Einfluss des O_2 druckes in der Einatmungshift auf die Alemtatigkeit des Menschen geprüft unter Konstanthultang des alveolarea CO_2 Druckes. *Arch. Ges. Physiol.* 267: 460–477, 1958.
38. Longobardo, G. S., N. S. Cherniack, and A. P. Fishman. Cheyne-Stokes breathing produced by a model of the human respiratory system. *J. Appl. Physiol.* 21: 1839–1846, 1966.
39. Lourenco, R. V., N. S. Chermack, J. F. Malm, and A. P. Fishman. Nervous output from the respiratory center during obstructed breathing. *J. Appl. Physiol.* 21: 527–533, 1966.
40. Middendorf, T., H. H. Loeschcke, and G. Ewald. Mathematische Analyse des Respirations systems. *Kybernetik* 10: 203–219, 1972.
41. Milhorn, H. T., Jr., and A. C. Guyton. An analog computer analysis of Cheyne-Stokes breathing. *J. Appl. Physiol.* 20: 328–338, 1965.
42. Milic-Emili, J., and J. M. Tyler. Relation between work output of respiratory muscles and end-tidal CO_2 tension. *J. Appl. Physiol.* 18: 497–504, 1963.
43. Mitchell, R. A., and A. J. Berger. Neural regulation of respiration. *Am. Rev. Respir. Dis.* 111: 206–224, 1976.
44. Mitchell, R. A., C. T. Carman, J. W. Severinghaus, B. W. Richardson, M. W. Singer, and S. Shnider. Stability of cerebrospinal fluid pH in chronic acid-base disturbances in blood. *J. Appl. Physiol.* 20: 443–552, 1965.
45. Mitchell, R. A., H. H. Loeschcke, J. W. Severinghaus, B. W. Richardson, and W. H. Massion. Regions of respiratory chemosensitivity on the surface of the medulla. *Ann. N.Y. Acad. Sci.* 109: 661–681, 1963.
46. Mitchell, R. A., and M. M. Singer. Respiration and cerebrospinal fluid pH in metabolic acidosis and alkalosis. *J. Appl. Physiol.* 20: 905–911, 1965.
47. Nielsen, M., and H. Smith. Studies on the regulation of respiration in acute hypoxia. *Acta Physiol. Scand.* 24: 293–313, 1951.
48. Pappenheimer, J. R., V. Fencl, S. R. Heisey, and D. Held. Role of cerebral fluids in control of respiration as studied in unanesthetized goats. *Am. J. Physiol.* 208: 436–450, 1965.
49. Priban, I. P., and W. F. Fincham. Self-adaptive control and the respiratory system. *Nature* 208: 339–343, 1965.
50. Rebuck, A. S., and E. J. M. Campbell. Clinical method for assessing the ventilatory response to hypoxia. *Am. Rev. Respir. Dis.* 109: 345–350, 1974.
51. Severinghaus, J. W. Proposed standard determination of ventilatory responses to hypoxia and hypercapnia in man. *Chest* 1977. (*In press.*)
52. von Euler, C. Proprioceptive control in respiration. In: *Nobel Symposium 1, Muscular Afferents and Motor Control.* Stockholm, Sweden: Almquist and Wiksell, 1966.
53. von Euler, C. The role of proprioceptive afferents in the control of respiratory muscle. *Acta Neurobiol. Exp (Warsz)* 33: 329–341, 1973.

54. Weil, J. V., E. Byrne-Quinn, I. E. Sodol, W. O. Friesen, B. Underhill, G. F. Filley, and R. F. Grover. Hypoxic ventilatory drive in normal man. *J. Clin. Invest.* **49**: 1061–1072, 1970.
55. Whitelaw, W. A., J. P. Derenne, and J. Milic-Emili. Occlusion pressure as a measure of respiratory center output in conscious man. *Respir. Physiol.* **23**: 181–199, 1975.
56. Widdicombe, J. G. Reflex control of breathing. In: *MTP International Review of Science, Physiology*, Series 1, *Respiratory Physiology*, Vol. 2. Edited by J. G. Widdicombe. London: Thornton Butterworth Ltd., 1974, pp. 273–301.
57. Wyman, R. J. Neural generation of the breathing rhythm. *Ann. Rev. Physiol.* **39**: 417–448, 1977.
58. Yamamoto, W. S., and M. W. Edwards, Jr. Homeostasis of carbon dioxide during intravenous infusion of carbon dioxide. *J. Appl. Physiol.* **15**: 807–818, 1960.
59. Yamashiro, S. M., J. A. Daubenspeck, T. N. Lauritsen, and F. S. Grodins. Total work rate of breathing optimization in CO_2 inhalation and exercise. *J. Appl. Physiol.* **38**: 702–709, 1975.

Index

Acid-base balance, 95–107
  chemical mechanisms, 95–103
  disturbances, 103–106
    metabolic, 103–104
    respiratory, 105–106
Acid or base excess of blood, 101–103
Adult respiratory distress syndrome (ARDS), 83
Airway closure, 38–44
Airway compression, 39
Airway model, 46, 47, 48t, 49t
Alkalemia, 111
Alveolar air, 4, 14, 47, 51t, 52–54, 58–60
Alveolar collapse, 35, 36
Alveolar diagram, 59
Alveolar ducts, 46–47, 48t, 49t
Alveolar fraction, 52–54, 56–57
Alveolar gas sampling, 53
Alveolar instability, 35–36
Alveolar pressure, 12–13, 20–22, 30–32
Alveolar space, 52–57
Alveoli, 47, 48t, 49t
Aortic bodies, 121
Apnea, 19
Apneustic breathing, 129
Apneustic center, 128
Arousal, 117, 123
Ataxic breathing, 131
Atelectasis, 83

Base excess, 101–103

Bends (decompression sickness), 91
Bert, Paul, 91, 94
Berylliosis, 69
Bicarbonate-pH acid-base diagram, 97–99
Block diagram, 6–7, 108–14, 117, 118
Blood-brain barrier, 122
Blood gases, 61–65
  bound, 61
    bicarbonate, 61
    carbamate, 61
    oxyhemoglobin, 61
  dissociation curves, 63–65
  free, 61
  normal values, 62t
Body plethysmograph, 12, 25
Bohr effect, 64
Bohr formulas, 52–57
Boyle, Robert, 9
Brain stem transection, 129–31
Breathing patterns, 125, 129, 131–35
Breuer, Joseph, 129, 131, 133, 138
Bronchi, 47, 48t
Bronchial circulation, 46–47, 48, 50
Bronchiectasis, 83, 84
Bronchioles, 46, 47, 48t
BTPS, 10, 58
Buffering, 95–107
  active (physiological), 103–106
  passive (chemical), 95–103
Buffering capacity, 99
Buffers, 95–107

Buffers (**Cont.**)
  blood, 97–103
    titration, 101–103
    definition and quantitation, 95–97

CO_2-O_2 diagram, 59
CO_2 dissociation (absorption) curve, 63–64
CO_2-O_2 interaction, 117–21
CO_2 response curve, 119–21, 123
CO_2 tension, P_{CO_2}, 4, 5, 49, 50, 51t, 52, 57–60, 61–65, 70–71, 88–90
  alveolar, $P_{A_{CO_2}}$, 4, 5, 50, 51t, 57–60
  arterial, $P_{a_{CO_2}}$, 4, 5, 50, 51t, 61–65
  effective, $P_{e_{CO_2}}$, 49, 50, 51t, 57–60
  effective-arterial gradient, $P_{e_{CO_2}}$-$P_{a_{CO_2}}$, 52, 70, 71
  end capillary, $P_{e_{CO_2}}$, 4, 5, 49, 50, 51t
  expired, $P_{E_{CO_2}}$, 4, 5, 50, 51t
  inspired, $P_{I_{CO_2}}$, 4, 5, 50, 51t
  mixed venous, $P_{V_{CO_2}}$, 4, 5, 50, 51t, 61–65
  tissue, $P_{T_{CO_2}}$, 88–90
  tracheal, $P_{i_{CO_2}}$, 51t
Carbon monoxide, 69
Carbonic anhydrase, 67
Cardiac output, 5
Cardiovascular system, 3
Carotid bodies, 121, 122
Central expiratory activity (CEA), 128
Central inspiratory activity or excitation (CIA or CIE), 128, 133
Central pattern generator, CPG, 127
Cerebrospinal fluid, CSF, 122
Chemoreceptors, 117
  central, 117
  peripheral, 117
Cheyne-Stokes breathing, 136
Chloride shift, 98
Chronic obstructive lung disease, COLD, 37, 69–70, 83
Clark, F. J., 131–33, 138
Clark-von Euler model, 131–33
Closed-loop, 109
Closing volume, 38, 40–44
Comparator, 110
Compensatory responses, 114
Compliance, 22–24, 30–37
  dynamic, 36–37
  lung, 30–34
  lung-thorax, 23
  static, 23–24, 30–34
  thorax, 30–34

Conductive airway, 52–54
Conjugate base, 95–96
Control of breathing, 108–41
  chemical, 110–25
  neural, 125–37
Control system, 108–10
Controlled system, 109
Controller gain, 123
Controller laws, 109–10
  basic chemostat, 113–14
  CO_2-O_2 interaction, 117–21
  cycle controller, 130, 131–35
  in exercise, 114–17
  integral, 110
  Lloyd equation, 122
  proportional, 110
Controller output, 123–24
Controller sensitivity, 123–24
Controlling signal, 110
Controlling system, 109
Cortical radiation, 117
Corticospinal tracts, 128
Cournand, André, 78, 85
Critical velocity, 27
Cunningham, D. J. C., 119–21, 131, 138

Dalton's law, 9
Dead space, 4, 46–48, 50, 51t, 52–57
  alveolar, 47–48, 50, 51t, 54–57
  conductive, 47–48, 50, 51t, 52–54
  parallel, 56
  physiological, 53, 57
  series, 56
  total, 57
  virtual, 54
Decompression sickness, 91
Desired value, 109
Diffusion, 3, 65–70, 86–94
  capacity, DO_2, 65, 69–70
  dysequilibrium, 66–68
  Fick's law, 65
  Krogh cylinder model, 86–88
  pulmonary, 3, 65–70
  tissue, 3, 86–94
Diffusion capacity, 65, 69–70
Dipalmitoyl lecithin, 35–36
Diving, 91–94
Dorsal respiratory group, 127
Dynamic compliance, 36–37
Dynamic resistance, 36–37
Dynamics of breathing, 20–37

Effective alveolar fraction, 54–57
Effective fraction, 54–57
Effective stimuli, 121–22
Elastic properties, 22–24, 30–37
  lung, 30–34
  lung-thorax, 23

INDEX   145

thorax, 30–34
Electromyograms, 124
Emphysema, 37, 69–70, 83
End-capillary blood, 4, 5, 49, 50, 51t, 57, 66–68
Equation of motion, 21–23
Ergoreceptors, 117, 123
Error signal, 109
Esophageal pressure, 32
Eupnea, 19
Exercise hyperpnea, 114–17
Expanded chemostat, 125, 126
Expiratory duration, T_E, 132

Feedback control system, 108–10
Fick's law, 65, 71
Flow volume curve, 38–40
Forced expiratory volume (FEV_1), 37
Function tests, pulmonary mechanics, 37–44
Functional residual capacity, FRC, 18

Gain coefficients, 123
Gas-blood matching, analysis of, 57–60, 71–76, 76–84
  continuous distribution model, 80–82
  exchange in single alveolus, 57–60, 71–76
  nonuniform $\dot{V}_e/\dot{Q}_e$ ratios, 76–84
  in normal man, 76–77
  three-compartment model, 77–80
Gas exchanger, 46–85, 86–94
  pulmonary, 46–85
    blood phase, 61–65
    blood-gas matching, 71–82
    disturbances of, 83–84
    gas phase, 52–60
    gas-blood gradients, 70–71
    ventilation/perfusion ratio, 71–82
  tissue, 86–94
    CO_2 exchange, 88–90
    decompression sickness, 90–94
    Krogh diffusion model, 86–88
    N_2 exchange, 90–94
    O_2 exchange, 86–88
    perfusion limited exchange, 89–90
Gas laws, 8–16
Gray, John S., v, 7, 104, 110, 111, 114, 120, 125, 138

Haldane alveolar sample, 53
Haldane decompression schedule, 91–94
Haldane effect, 64, 98
Hamburger shift, 98
Hasselbalch, K. A., 96
Henderson equation, 96
Henderson, L. J., 96, 106
Henderson-Hasselbalch equation, 96

Henry's law, 11
Hering, Ewald, 129, 131, 133, 139
Hering-Breuer reflex, 129, 131, 133
Hey, L. N., 131
Hey plot, 131, 132, 134
Heymans, C. J. F., 121
Homeostasis, 2, 95
Hyalin membrane disease, 36
Hypercapnia, 59–60, 110
Hyperoxia, 59–60, 111
Hyperpnea, 19
Hyperventilation, 59–60, 100–101
Hypocapnia, 59–60, 111
Hypoventilation, 59–60, 76, 100–101
Hypoxia, 60, 110, 114

Ideal exchanger, 71, 77–80
Ideal gas, 8
Inert gas exchange, 80–82, 90–94
Information flow, 117
Inspiratory duration, T_I, 132
Inspiratory off-switch, 128–31, 132–35
Inspiratory spinal cells (IS), 133
Inspiratory vagal cells (IV), 133
Involuntary (automatic) control of breathing, 127–31
Irritant receptors, 135

J-receptors, 135

Krogh, August, 86–88, 94
Krogh cylinder, 86–88
Krogh's hypothesis, 87

Lambertsen, C. J., 7, 122, 139
Laminar flow, 26–27
Laminar flow "wash-out," 54
Laplace's law, 35
Lloyd, B. B., 119–21, 122–23, 131, 139
Lung volumes, 17–18
  derived, 18
    functional residual capacity (FRC), 18
    inspiratory capacity, 18
    total lung capacity, 18, 38
    vital capacity, 18
  primary, 17–18
    expiratory reserve, 18
    inspiratory reserve, 18
    residual, 18
    tidal, 17, 18

Mass action law, 95–96
Material flow, 6, 117
Maximum expiratory flow, 37–40
Mechanics of breathing, 17–45
Medullary respiratory centers, 127–28
Medullary switch, 128–31, 132–35

Metabolic acidosis, 103–104
Metabolic alkalosis, 103–104
Metabolic hyperpnea, 114–17
Metabolic servomechanism, 2–3, 6–7, 108, 114–17, 118
Metabolic system, 4
Metaboloreceptors, 123
Muscle driving pressure, $P_{M(t)}$, 22, 28–29, 124

Negative feedback, 108–10
Neural circuitry, control of breathing, 127–31
Nielsen, M., 119–20, 140
Nonbicarbonate buffer curve, 99–101
Nucleus ambiguus, 127
Nucleus parabrachialis, NPB, 128
Nucleus reticularis gigantocellularis, 128
Nucleus reticularis ventralis, 128
Nucleus retroambigualis, 127

Obstructive lung disease, 37, 69–70, 83
Occlusion pressure, P_{100}, 124
Operating point, 110
Oxford fan, 120–21
Oxygen capacity, 61, 63
Oxygen content, 63
Oxygen dissociation curve, 63–65
  P_{50}, 65
Oxygen saturation, 63
O_2 tension, P_{O_2}, 4, 5, 49, 50, 51t, 52, 57–60, 61–65, 70–71, 88–90
  alveolar, $P_{A_{O_2}}$, 4, 5, 50, 51t, 57–60
  arterial, $P_{a_{O_2}}$, 4, 5, 50, 51t, 61–65
  effective, $P_{e_{O_2}}$, 49, 50, 51t, 57–60
  effective-arterial gradient, $P_{e_{O_2}}$-$P_{a_{O_2}}$, 52, 70–71
  end capillary, $P_{e_{CO_2}}$, 4, 5, 49, 50, 51t
  expired, $P_{E_{O_2}}$, 4, 5, 50, 51t
  inspired, $P_{I_{O_2}}$, 4, 5, 50, 51t
  mixed venous, $P_{V_{O_2}}$, 4, 5, 50, 51t, 61–65
  tissue, $P_{T_{O_2}}$, 86–88
  tracheal, $P_{i_{O_2}}$, 50, 51t
Oxygen tension gradient in tissue, 86–88
  brain, 88
  myocardium, 88

Pacemaker cells, 135
Pappenheimer, J. R., 122, 140
Parabolic velocity profile, 26–27
Partition coefficient, 81

P_e-P_a gradients, 70–71
Periodic breathing, 136
Peripheral receptors, 121–23
Phrenic neurograms, 124
Physiological dead space, 54–57
  alveolar, 54–56
  conductive, 54
  total, 57
Plant, 109, 111–13
Plant law, 111–13
Pleural pressure, 30–32
Pneumotachogram, 20
Pneumotachograph, PTG, 20
Pneumotaxic center, 128–31
Pneumothorax, 32
Poiseuille's law, 27
Pressure-volume curves, 23, 30, 32–34
Protein buffer line, 99–101
Pulmonary elasticity, 23, 32–34
Pulmonary ventilation, 3, 4–6, 19, 46–60, 108–41
  alveolar, 50, 51t, 52–54
  control of, 6–7, 108–41
  dead space, 50, 51t, 54–57
  effective, 50, 51t, 54–57
  expired, 50, 51t
  inspired, 50, 51t, 52

Ramp generator, 133–35
Reaction rates, 66–69
Receptor sites, 121–23, 135–37
Receptors, 121–23, 128–29, 135–37
  chemo-, 121–23
    central, 121–22
    peripheral, 121
  ergo-, 117, 123
  irritant, 135, 137
  J-, 135, 137
  metabolo-, 117, 123
  stretch, 128–29
Regulation, 2, 6–7, 95, 108–10
Relaxation pressure-volume curves, 23, 30–34
Relman, A. S., 103
Residual volume, 18, 38
Resistive load, 124
  effect on CO_2 response curve, 124
Resistive properties, 24–28, 36–37, 38–40
Respiratory acidosis, 99, 105
Respiratory alkalosis, 99, 105
Respiratory bronchioles, 47, 48t
Respiratory centers, 127–31
Respiratory chemostat, 110–17
  block diagram, 112
  buffer component, 112–13
  controller law, 113–14
  in exercise, 114–17
  plant laws, 111–13

Respiratory compensation line, 104, 105, 106
Respiratory compensation pathway, 104, 105, 106
Respiratory controller output, choice of, 123–24
Respiratory cycle, 18–20, 125–35
Respiratory exchange ratio (R), 4–6
Respiratory quotient (RQ), 4–6
Respiratory regulation equations, 112–13, 117, 119, 122
Respiratory work, 29–30, 124
 elastic, 29
 measure of controller output, 124
 negative, 30
 resistive, 29
 useful, 30
Respiratory zone model, 49t
Reynolds number, 27
Rohrer, Fritz, 20, 45

Saline-filled lungs, elastic properties of, 33–34
Schwartz, W. B., 103, 107
Self-oscillator, 127
Servomechanism, 2–3, 108–10, 114–17, 118
Servomechanism theory, 3, 108–10
Set point, 110
Shock lung, 83
Shunt, 4, 46–51, 70–71, 75–76, 77–80
 alveolar, 48, 50, 51t, 70–71, 75–76, 77–80
 conductive, 48, 50, 51t
Siggaard-Andersen, O., 101, 107
Siggaard-Andersen formula for base excess, 101
Smith, H., 119–20
Solitary tract, nucleus of, 127–28
Solubility coefficients, 11
Spirogram, 18–20
Spirometer, 17–20
Stability of alveoli, 35, 36
Stage decompression, 91–94
Standard atmosphere, 13t
Standard bicarbonate content of true plasma, $[BHCO_3]_{7.40}$, 103
Steady-state error, 111, 116
STPD, 58
Stretch receptors, 128–29
Surface tension, 35–36
Surfactant, 35–36
System law, 109
Systems analysis, 1, 108–10

Tachypnea, 20
Thews, G., 88, 94
Thoracic gas volume, measurement of, 12

Tidal volume, 17–18
Tissue oxygen pressure, 86–88
Tonic CO_2 drive, 133–35, 136
Total lung capacity, 38
Trachea, 46, 47
Tracheal air, 49, 51t
Transpulmonary pressure, 31–32
Transthoracic pressure, 31–32
True plasma, 98
Turbulent flow, 26–28

Unit process, 1, 3–5, 109, 125
Unstressed volume, 23, 30–32, 34
 lung, 30–32, 34
 lung-thorax, 23
 thorax, 30–32, 34

Vagal stretch reflex, 128–29, 131–35
Van Slyke blood gas analyzer, 63
Variable, 109
 dependent, 109
 independent, 109
 regulated, 109
Venous admixture, 4, 46–51, 70–71, 77–80, 83–84
Ventilation, 3, 4–7, 19, 46–60, 108–41
 alveolar, 50, 51t, 52–54
 capacity, 19
 control of, 6–7, 108–41
 dead space, 50, 51t, 54–57
 effective, 50, 51t, 54–57
 expired, 50, 51t
 inspired, 50, 51t, 52
Ventilation capacity, 19
Ventilation/perfusion ratio ($\dot{V}_e/\dot{Q}_e$), 70–82
Ventilatory apparatus, 3, 17–45, 123
Ventilatory equivalent, 59–60
Ventilatory reserve, 19–20
Ventilatory response, 114–21
 to CO_2, 115, 117–21
 to exercise, 114–17
 to metabolic acid-base disturbances, 116
 to oxygen lack, 115, 117–21
Ventral respiratory group, 127
Virtual dead space, 54
Virtual volumes, 53
Viscosity, 21–23, 26–28
 dynamic, 26–27
 kinematic, 28
Vital capacity, 18
Volume-time threshold, 131–35
Voluntary control of breathing, 128–29, 130, 131
Von Euler, C., 131–35, 140

Wagner, P. D., 80, 85

Water vapor, 9–11
Weibel, E. R., 47, 48t, 49t, 52, 85
Work of breathing, 29–30, 124
　elastic, 29
　measure of controller-output, 124
　negative, 30
　resistive, 29
　useful, 30

Xenon, 40–41, 76–77
　measurement of closing volume, 40–41
　measurement of $\dot{V}/\dot{Q}$ nonuniformity, 76–77

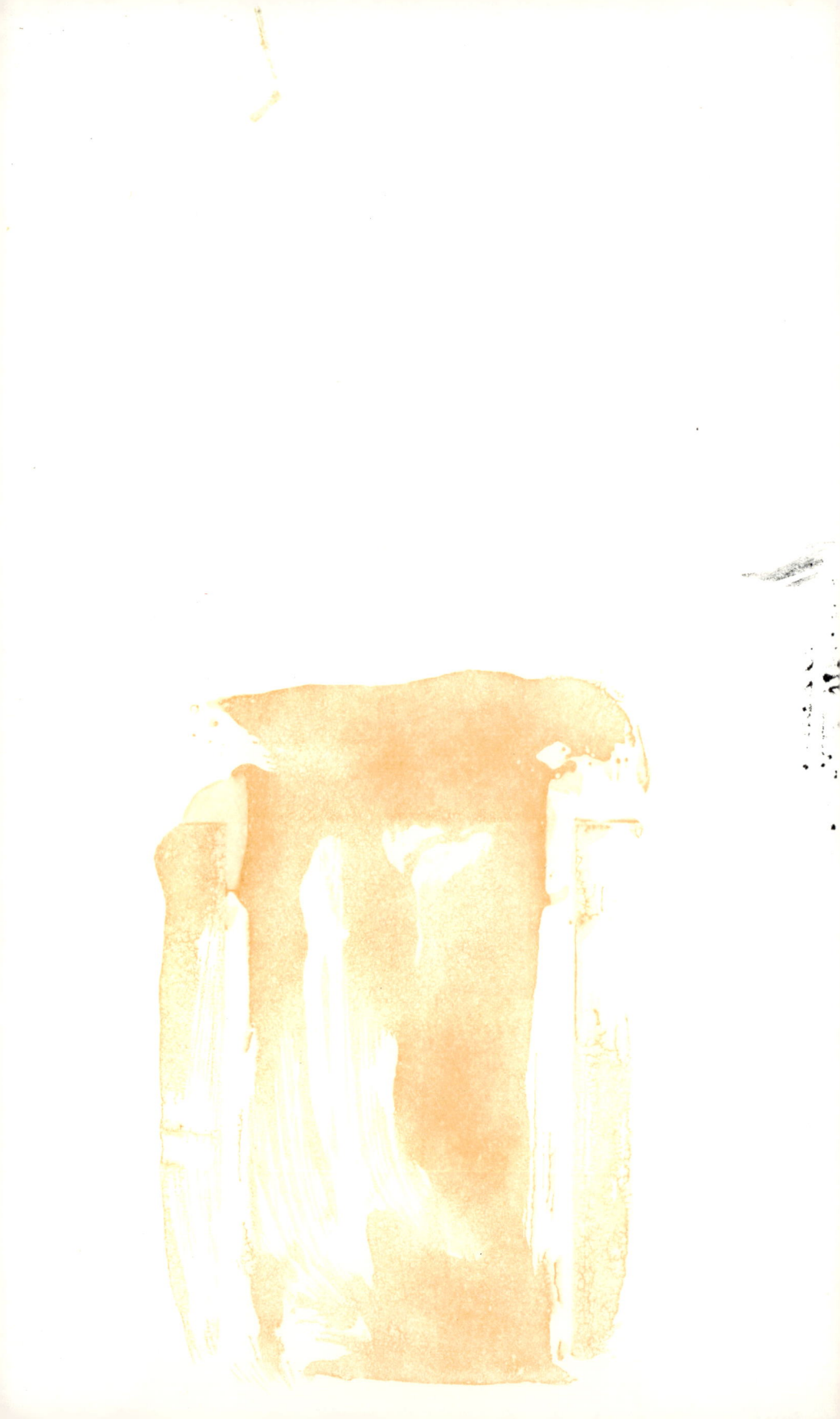